Running Out of Gas

For the runners I call grizzled veterans...
And everyone who hopes to be one.

SCOTT LUDWIG

RUNNING
OUT
OF GAS

A LIFELONG RUNNER'S
TAKE ON SLOWING DOWN

Meyer & Meyer Sport

British Library Cataloguing in Publication Data
A catalogue record for this book is available from the British Library

Running Out of Gas
A Lifelong Runner's Take on Slowing Down
Maidenhead: Meyer & Meyer Sport (UK) Ltd., 2018
ISBN: 978-1-78255-127-0

© 2018 by Meyer & Meyer Sport (UK) Ltd.
Aachen, Auckland, Beirut, Cairo, Cape Town, Dubai, Hägendorf, Hong Kong, Indianapolis,
Manila, New Delhi, Singapore, Sydney, Tehran, Vienna

Member of the World Sports Publishers' Association (WSPA)
Printed by Seaway Printing
ISBN: 978-1-78255-127-0
Email: info@m-m-sports.com
www.m-m-sports.com

CONTENTS

2014 – A Change of Direction

2015 – Going Out With Both Barrels Blazing

2016 – Serious As a Heart Attack

2017 – Well Past the Finish Line

FOREWORD

It's inevitable that all runners who have been pounding the pavement for a very long time will eventually slow down. Having run every day since November 30, 1978, I am certainly one of those who fall into this category.

Fortunately for me, I've had my good friend and running partner, Al Barker—almost 10 years my senior—preparing me for the inevitable for quite some time. Al has taken the time to walk me (both literally and figuratively) through the reality of slowing down with age gracefully so that when the moment finally arrived—and by all means it has definitely arrived—I would be prepared. Now that I can no longer run a single mile in the pace I ran 26 of them when I set my marathon best many years ago, I can say that Al has done a great job. I'm totally fine with it.

So where does that leave me now? I'd like to think that places me clearly among the ranks of what I've always referred to as the "grizzled veterans." The kind of runner you look to for the wisdom and insight they gained from their many years and miles on the roads or trails.

I'm here to tell you I've got plenty of both. Well, the miles for sure; the wisdom and insight—you be the judge. Some of it is pretty sound and sensible; then again, some is not. As you will soon learn, I'm definitely a "do as I say, not as I do" type of runner. I can dole out pretty good advice, but I'll be damned if I'm able to follow it.

Maybe the best example I can offer is when I ran the Western States Endurance Run in 2006, a 100-mile race through the

Sierra Nevada mountain range in California. After running 62 miles and for more than 16 hours with my shoes and socks soaking wet, courtesy of traversing through an assortment of snow, melting snow, and overflowing streams, I stopped at an aid station to have my feet examined. A medic removed my shoes and socks and advised me to pull myself from the race because the balls of both of my feet were split wide open, and there was a pretty good chance of infection, not to mention the possible loss of one or both feet if I kept running. I looked him squarely in the eyes and said the first and only thing that crossed my mind: "Got any duct tape?"

So what you are about to read is my advice to you, dear runner. Listen to what I have to say, but be warned, it might be best to shy away from most of the things I've done.

In other words, do as I say, not as I do. In the long run you'll be better off. Trust me.

PROLOGUE

When I began writing this book in February 2013, I had already been running every other day for more than 34 years, accumulating 130,000-pluse miles and completing over 800 races. I provide this information to give you the foundation for what you are about to read.

2013

PASSING
THE TORCH

SPECIAL DAY

FEBRUARY 2013

Today was a special day.

I ran with my good friend Al this morning for maybe the 2,000th time. Somewhere between the fifth and sixth mile of our 10-mile run, I reached my 130,000th lifetime mile.

Al and I have been running together for almost 20 years. We both started running during the "Running Boom" of the 1970's, and neither one of us has had the inclination or desire to stop.

We've run races—mostly marathons—in states all across the United States. Florida (Tallahassee, Jacksonville, Five Points of Life), Massachusetts (Boston), Minnesota (Grandma's), Alabama (Vulcan, Mercedes), Virginia (Shamrock), North Carolina (Grandfather Mountain), South Carolina (Columbia), Nevada (Las Vegas), Utah (St. George), Illinois (Chicago), and Georgia (Atlanta, Tybee Island, Callaway Gardens, Chickamauga Battlefield, Macon, Albany, Museum of Aviation, and Soldiers). We've competed in ultras in some of the most amazing places on the planet, including the Sierra Nevada Mountain Range and Death Valley. We also managed an embarrassing last-place finish in an ultra at Oak Mountain (Alabama) several years ago. Al and I are cut from the same cloth: the cloth indicating you're going to be a lousy trail runner.

If you ever want to know more about Al, I've written about him in one way or another in all of the books I've written about running.

In fact, one of my books, *In It for the Long Run: A Decade With the Darkside Running Club* has an entire chapter devoted to Al.

Over the years and the miles, Al and I have pretty much solved every problem known to humanity. We've dissected our respective physical ailments thousands of times. We've psychoanalyzed every last one of our friends, foes, and family members. We've met every crisis in both of our lives head on, and we know deep down inside we've figured out a way for things to work out in the end. Hell, we've even figured out how to obtain world peace; now if only someone would ask us.

Today was a special day, but not because I ran my 130,000th mile. Today was a special day because, after running a cumulative 70-plus years and 200,000-plus miles, Al and I still have the health and the desire to run 10 miles at 5:30 a.m. on a bitterly cold and dark Saturday morning…and appreciate every second of it.

Footnote: I posted this story on my Facebook page. I received a great deal of comments but one in particular stood out:

I appreciate you, your heart—for running and for grand parenting!—and your motivation, inspiration, and encouragement—all of which you have given to many through the years.

I've spent my entire running career doing everything in my power to promote the sport, and my grandson Krischan means the world to me. That being said, I sent a note to the author and told her it was one of the nicest things anyone has ever said to me. I have never been more sincere in my life. *Stellise—one more time, thank you.*

ASPHALT THERAPY

FEBRUARY 2013

Many of my friends think I've been running with Al Barker longer than anyone else. My friends would be wrong. The truth of the matter is I've been running with Valerie longer.

Val and I started running together in early fall of 1993. Her goal was to qualify for the Boston Marathon. We circled Thanksgiving Day on our calendars, the (then) traditional day of the Atlanta Marathon. We trained hard for several months, and on one incredible Thursday, Val ran a sensational race and qualified to run Boston the following April; I ran alongside as her pacer. At the finish line Al came over to congratulate Val...and he and I met for the very first time. The three of us began running together every Sunday; 20 miles was our minimum. Occasionally we'd run 25, 30, even 40 miles depending on what we were training for. We began running marathons and ultras (races longer than 26.2 miles) all over the country. There was an article about the three of us in a running publication that covered the sport in the southeast. The article was appropriately titled, *An Enduring Friendship.*

Last May, Val, Susan, and I began running from Val's property every Sunday morning in beautiful Senoia, Georgia. If you're a fan of the hit television series *The Walking Dead* you would recognize some of the scenery we have the privilege of enjoying every week on our long runs along the rolling asphalt country roads of Senoia (or Woodbury for you *Walking Dead* fans). In fact, I am so enamored with the area that in six weeks I will be putting on The Running Dead Ultra, a 42.6-mile race along many of the roads we've explored these past nine months (you'll hear more about it later). The race will start and finish in front of Val's property.

This morning, however, Susan didn't show up for our run. I've been running with Susan for over 10 years, and she has *always* shown up, even on the couple of days when she should have stayed in bed (she, like Val, Al, and me, is a trooper when it comes to our running commitments). If Susan is running late she'll always send a text message or email. However, today was different. Not only because of Susan's inexplicable absence, but also because this morning brought the thickest, densest fog I've ever seen in my life. To say I was worried about her would be an understatement. No Susan, no *word* from Susan, and fog as thick as pea soup—a pea soup that Susan had to drive over 40 miles through to meet up with us. I called her cell phone but could only leave a message when she didn't answer.

Val and I waited 30 minutes for Susan before we headed out for our run. I told Val how worried I was about Susan; she assured me Susan would be just fine and probably just overslept. I told Val I was worried about the used car I helped my son Justin buy the day before: the test drive, the sale, and everything associated with the car went so well that I kept hearing "if it seems too good to be true it probably is" in my mind. Val said the car would be just fine, and I was wasting my time worrying about it; whatever will be will be and all.

It wasn't too long before we found ourselves switching roles. Val was now on the couch, unloading her recent fears and anxieties, and I was in the big leather chair offering reassurance and guidance. To say our run was a highlight reel for the *Doctor Phil Show* wouldn't have been far from the truth.

But that's how it is every Sunday on our long, relaxing runs along the asphalt country roads of Senoia. Call it what you will: therapy, counseling, friendly advice, telling one another what we want, no, *need* to hear, or simply talking to make the miles pass by quicker.

Regardless of what you might call it, we've been doing it for over 20 years, and I'll be the first to tell you it *works*.

After Val and I finished our run, I had a message on my cell phone from Susan. She woke up very, very sick in the middle of the night and sent me an email shortly after midnight saying Val and I should go on without her. However, her email never made it to me *(I told you the fog was thick!)*. But Val was right: Susan was just fine. I now had faith she was right about Justin's car as well.

I love running with my friends for many reasons. It allows us to catch up with one another's lives. It provides us the opportunity to share our hopes and dreams, our problems and fears. It makes running fun.

Most of all, I love running with my friends simply because they are, in the truest sense of the word, my friends.

RESTRAINT

MARCH 2013

I ran the Comrades Marathon in South Africa in 2011. It was my 50th ultramarathon, and I thought that would be a nice round number to round out my ultramarathon career.

I ran the Honolulu Marathon in 2012. It was my 200th marathon, and I thought that would be a nice round number to complete my marathon career.

Why put an end to something I enjoy doing? It all comes down to a matter of health; or in my case, the lack thereof. I haven't been anywhere near 100% physically since I ran 62 miles in the Sierra Nevada mountains in the summer of 2004. The race, the Western States Endurance Run, was my first attempt at running 100 miles on trails. As evidenced by the 62 miles I mentioned earlier, I didn't finish the race. I did, however, manage to lay the foundation for subsequent damage to my body should I ever try something as stupid as Western States again; after all I'm a "flatland runner" and would much prefer running on asphalt roads rather than treacherous mountain trails.

The damage was complete when I returned to the same race again two years later. This time I managed to finish the race (in last place; but I finished, dammit!). I also managed to put the finishing touches to the foundation I laid two years prior. A bulging disk in my lower back led to numbness in my right leg that led to circulation problems that led to…well, let's just say the list goes on and on.

I've enjoyed running since I began in the summer of 1978, but I'll be the first to admit every run since the summer of 2006 has been somewhat of a challenge. 2012 was a difficult year, as it was my goal to complete 15 marathons during the year to finish with number 200 in Honolulu in December. Cindy met me at the finish line in Honolulu with a kiss and a question: "How does it feel to be finished running marathons?" (Coming full circle: Cindy gave me a kiss and wished me luck as I began my first marathon in Gainesville, Florida, almost 34 years prior.) I surprised myself with my answer: "Fantastic; I am so glad it's over." Until that very moment, I could never have imagined having those feelings.

For over three decades I had been running marathons, enjoying each and every step. Crossing the finish line was always one of the best feelings I've ever experienced...until the last three or four times. The thrill was gone. It was time to call it quits. No looking back.

So today I ran in a friend's race in Cumming, Georgia: The Stroll in Central Park 12-Hour Run. I told my friend I would come up and run for a few hours but would have to leave as I was meeting Cindy in Atlanta; we were running the Georgia Half Marathon the next morning. I also didn't want to run 26.2 miles or more and ruin my nice round numbers: 50 and 200.

The course was a 1.03-mile loop. I ran an easy pace and decided I would have to be finished running by 1:00 p.m. to meet Cindy (the race started at 8:00 a.m.). As I was finishing my 25th loop around 12:45 p.m., I told the scorer I was finished for the day. I was content with my 25.75 miles. The scorer was a friend of mine and encouraged me to run "one more loop" to finish a marathon (26.2 miles). Another friend said to run enough laps to qualify my run as an official 50-kilometer (31-mile) ultramarathon. I reminded them both that I was finished with both marathons and ultramarathons. I said if I ran a marathon today I would then have 201, and being the anal person I am that would require me to run enough marathons to get to the next round number: 210. And if I were to finish 210 marathons I would feel obligated to get to the *next* round number: 300. (Note: When I say I'm an anal person, I'm not exaggerating. Not in the least.) They both understood that I was in no way, shape, or form joking and as such immediately backed off from encouraging me to run any farther.

Before I left I asked my race director friend if by chance the course was actually one-point-oh-FIVE miles long, which would mean I had already run a full marathon. She assured me the loop was 1.03, preserving my record of 200 marathons. 200 even.

On the ride back to Atlanta, I was proud of myself for the restraint I had shown. Years ago—before the injuries of 2004 and 2006—the word was not even a part of my vocabulary.

At this stage of my life, restraint is very much in my vocabulary, especially if I want to preserve what's left of my health. I owe that much to my grandson (and any future grandchildren I may be blessed with).

BIG BUSINESS IS RUINING RUNNING

MARCH 2013

I mentioned running in the Stroll in Central Park 12-Hour Run several days ago. I enjoy races of this nature: low key, nice course, simple logistics, wonderful amenities for the runners, supportive and enthusiastic volunteers, and a race director who truly cares about the runners. And best of all, a reasonable entry fee.

There are also races I don't enjoy (Are you listening, New York City Marathon?): high profile, congested course, ridiculously difficult logistics, mediocre amenities, glamor-seeking volunteers, and a race director who cares primarily about making a profit. So expect to pay an exorbitant entry fee. (Close to $300 for the afore-referenced marathon!)

Road racing (particularly marathons) has turned into big business. Large corporations have taken over the world of marathoning (think ING, Rock 'N Roll, Nike). It's not uncommon to pay $150 or more to run 26.2 miles. If it's an out-of-town event, factor in the cost of transportation, meals, and hotels (which jack up their rates accordingly for their captive audience). If you're not a runner, the total expense to run a major marathon in a big city would astound you. If you *are* a runner, you know exactly what I'm talking about. I've gone on record in a couple of my other books saying you won't find me running the major marathons (New York City, Chicago, Los Angeles, etc.). Big business seems intent on taking the joy out of running, and I personally want no part of it.

Getting outfitted in a pair of shorts, a shirt, and a pair of running shoes shouldn't cost the same as a new washing machine, but it does. At the expo for the half marathon Cindy and I ran last Sunday (Cindy had a free entry for a survey about the prior year's race that I filled out in her name, while I registered early for a substantially reduced entry fee; otherwise we wouldn't have been there), a brand-new pair of Hoka running shoes were on sale for the reduced price of $149 (normally $159). A good pair of running shorts cost $40 or more; shirts may run slightly higher. Then expect to pay $15 or $20 for a really good pair of running socks. Factoring in any accessories (GPS, chronograph, sunglasses, cap, running belt, etc.) and BAM, you just paid for a washing machine. Speaking of washing machines, you can now purchase laundry detergent designed especially for washing running clothes. Anything to make a buck, right?

I admire, respect, and support those who promote running simply because they love the sport. I choose to ignore those who are simply out to make a dollar at the runner's expense and care nothing about the preservation of the sport.

When I finished the Stroll in Central Park last Saturday, the race director gave me a bottle of Blue Moon to drink once I got home and showered. When I finished the half marathon the next day, I grabbed a bottle of water from an unattended table just past the finish line.

You can probably guess which race I'll return to next year.

And it won't be because of the beer.

THE RUNNING DEAD
APRIL 2013

I have been hooked on the television series *The Walking Dead* since its debut. That it's filmed near and around my home in Peachtree City—mostly in the neighboring town of Senoia—makes it that much more appealing.

You see, I've been hooked on Senoia ever since I began doing my long runs there with Valerie last May. Val has a nice home with 40 acres along a lightly traveled asphalt country road, which happens to be my absolute favorite venue for running. On that very first run together 11 months ago, I told her I wanted to establish a long-distance footrace in Senoia because everything about the area was a perfect fit for an ultramarathon: beautiful scenery; long and rolling country roads virtually free of traffic; and her 40-acre farm that was just perfect for a post-race get-together. Added bonus: Plenty of room for the runners to park their cars!

We began running and exploring different 15- to 18-mile segments of the area each Sunday. Before long we started putting together a route for the race—approximately 40 miles in length that would include many of the locales, venues, and scenes from *The Walking Dead* television series.

I laid out a tentative course in my mind that included (you non-*Walking Dead* fans can skip to the paragraph after these bullet points if you'd like):

- Running right through the middle of "Woodbury" (Senoia),

allowing the runners to see (among other notable buildings in the television series) town hall and the Governor's residence.

- The mill scene in the last episode of season 2 where Rick proclaimed their small group was "no longer a democracy."

- The building where Rick and the Governor reached an "agreement" toward the end of season 3.

- The long road (Dead Oak) through the woods used for many of the driving scenes in the show.

The only problem was the course measured out to be 37 miles, a bit shy of the 41.3 miles I was looking for (66.6 kilometers; I thought 666 was a good number for a race with the word "dead" in its name). Eric, who will take over as race director next year, added a little loop along hilly Dolly Nixon Road at the end of the course, stretching the distance to 42.6 miles. Perfect, as far as I was concerned. Added bonus: Dolly Nixon was used to film the scene in season 3 when the backpacker tried (and failed) to hitch a ride with Rick and later in the episode was discovered to be zombie roadkill.

After a few emails, discussions, and one lone meeting with the good people of Senoia and Coweta County, the race was given the required blessing.

The plans for the race were set in motion when I named the race The Running Dead Ultra. I referred to it as 42.6 miles of Heaven …and Hell.

It was fun advertising for the race on Facebook. The posts for such an unusually-themed race came quite easily:

- There's only one rule for this event: Do not feed the zombies.

- If you're chased by zombies you don't have to be fast; just faster than the other runner.

- Smearing oneself with roadkill is a known zombie deterrent. It should be in ample supply all along the course.

There were officially 23 finishers in the inaugural event (for the history books, the "Male Survivor" was Steven Bothe and the "Female Survivor" was Kim Ruple; most races would call them the champions, but hey, this was *The Running Dead Ultra!*). Three runners failed to finish due to assorted physical ailments; they were listed in the official race results as "carnage."

As a bonus, runners enjoyed a trip through an old cemetery around the nine-mile mark along the course. One of our volunteers, decked out in full zombie makeup and wardrobe, hid behind one of the larger tombstones throughout the morning so she could greet each of the runners as they precariously ran along the cemetery, waiting to be scared.

We didn't let the runners down.

Good luck with the race next year, Eric. It has the potential to be one of the best of its kind in the country.

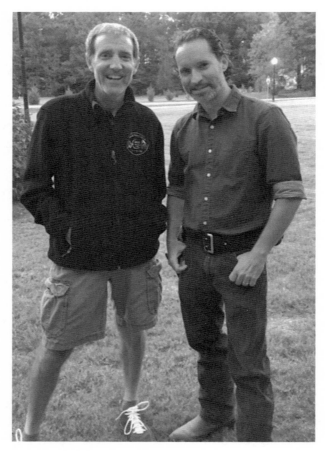

Scott and "Senoia Rick," who you may recognize from The Walking Dead

THE NEXT STEP

APRIL 2013

I would classify myself as an optimist. I always see the glass as half full. I find the silver lining. I look on the bright side of things.

That explains why I worked for more than 24 years for a company that did everything in its power to convert me to pessimism. Every day for over 24 years I would wake up with one thought in my head while driving into work: *"Today is going to be a good day."* However, the number of times I was right in those 24-plus years I can count on one hand. Have you ever had this thought during the course of your work day: *"If I knew it was going to be this bad I would have stayed in bed"?* If so, that pretty much describes every single day of those two-dozen years.

My current job is just the opposite. This December 1, I will have been with this company 10 years, and so far (knock on wood), I can count the number of *bad* days I've had on one hand. Perhaps "job karma" is rewarding me for my positive thinking those prior 24 years. *Good things come to he who waits. Patience is a virtue.*

Being an eternal optimist can be frustrating at times, particularly when it comes to my health. I've been battling various ailments and injuries since 2000 when I noticed numbness in my right thigh after running a marathon in Virginia Beach. Three years later after running a 135-mile race across Death Valley, I noticed a loss of quickness in my leg turnover. The next year I entered a 100-mile race through the mountains, only to drop out after 62 miles because both of my thighs felt like they had been sledgehammered; no, *jackhammered.* (Truth be known I had about as much business running in the mountains as an elephant has being on a skateboard. But I digress.) Two years later I returned to this same race intent on reaching the finish line. I finished the race…and my back hasn't been the same since after being subjected to more ups and downs than my body ever had been before.

I'm currently battling a bulging disk between my L-4 and L-5 vertebrae, most likely the result of the aforementioned 100 miles in the mountains. The effects of the bulging disk painfully manifest in various spots below my waist, apparently at the mercy of whichever direction the disk decides to bulge on any given day. Whatever the case—numbness in my leg, a sharp pain in my hip, stinging sensations in my calves—the pain has a dramatic effect on my running stride and almost always causes a significant amount of pain. But throughout these past 13-plus years I approach every run with the hope and perhaps expectation that my next step is going to be the one pain-free step I've been dying to take for a long, long time.

So far I haven't taken that step, but it doesn't darken my hopes and spirits that tomorrow will be the day I enjoy my first pain-free run in many, many years.

It truly is a double-edged sword: Experiencing the highs of hoping for the best and realizing the lows from realizing the disappointment. Such is the life of an optimist.

But then again, tomorrow is always another day.

PATRIOT'S DAY

APRIL 15, 2013

There was a time when I referred to the weekend of the Boston Marathon as my "Christmas in April." I consider myself very fortunate to have had the opportunity to run in the greatest foot-race in the world 12 times. When I first started running in 1978, I dreamed of one day lining up with the finest runners in the world in Hopkinton to run the fabled 26.2-mile route to Boston on Patriot's Day, a civic holiday in Massachusetts commemorating the anniversary of the Battle of Lexington and Concord, the first battles of the American Revolutionary War.

My first experience in Boston, perhaps my finest and certainly my most emotional, was in 1987. I can still vividly remember choking up as I ran the final stretch on Boyleston Street when the finish line banner was clearly within sight. To think that someone like me could run in this, the most prestigious marathon in the world, was indeed quite the thrill. I feel honored to have experienced that thrill 11 more times over the next 23 years, my last trip to Boston being in 2010. Ironically it was the first time Cindy made the trip with me. Although I didn't run particularly well in my Boston swan song, I was glad Cindy finally got to see me run beneath the most recognizable finish line banner on the planet.

I have some great memories of Boston. I lowered my personal best marathon time at my first Boston in 1987. I ran on the Atlanta Track Club Men's Masters Team several years, breaking three hours (my personal indicator of a solid effort) three times; my younger son Josh made the trip with me and was there to witness one of them. In 2003 I ran the course from the finish line to the start and then turned around and ran the race with everyone else to celebrate my 100th lifetime marathon. (Note: I was training for the Badwater Ultramarathon, a 135-mile event I would be running three months later.)

Nana, my grandmother on my mom's side and arguably my biggest supporter in running, passed away the weekend of the 1999 Boston Marathon. When I called my parents to tell them how I did after the race (it was my fastest Boston since my first one in 1987), my mom told me that Nana had passed away the day before, but she had waited until then to tell me because she knew Nana would not want me to be distracted from running well. Ironically, I was running in the pair of running shoes Nana had given me for Christmas four months earlier.

I had the privilege to meet many of my running idols during the Boston Marathon weekend: Bill Rodgers, Frank Shorter, and Bobbi Gibb, to name a few. I feel honored to have told Bobbi's story in my book *A Passion for Running: Portraits of the Everyday Runner.* Bobbi was the first woman to run the Boston Marathon and her story is remarkable. (I won't tell you about it here in hopes that you'll track down a copy of *Passion*!) I met Bobbi in person after the 2010 Boston Marathon (my 12th and in all probability my last) and will always remember what a genuinely nice and sincere woman she is.

I won't be running the Boston Marathon this year. Many of my friends will be, however, and for them I have one piece of advice:

Savor every step.

BOMBS ON BOYLSTON STREET

APRIL 16, 2013

By the time you are reading this, what happened yesterday in Boston will be a part of our country's history.

Bombs were detonated on Boylston Street near the finish line of the Boston Marathon. Clouds of death and devastating injury left an indelible, devastating mark on one of the greatest celebrations of life, health, and camaraderie in the world.

Many of my friends and running club members competed at the Boston Marathon yesterday. Thankfully all of them are safe; some perhaps not so sound. Throughout the afternoon, I saw Facebook posts from their family members and other friends indicating they were unharmed. All except one: My very close friend Gary from Tallahassee. I texted him and left a message on his cell phone asking if he was OK, only to learn that the people in Boston were asked not to use their cell phones for fear of detonating other bombs (if there were indeed other bombs). I called his wife Peg who was back home in Tallahassee; I had to leave a message there as well.

Twenty minutes passed before Gary returned my call. He had finished his marathon less than 15 minutes before the bombs exploded and was about half a mile away from the finish line when it happened. Everyone near him was in the dark about what had happened back at the finish line, police and race officials included.

I had the same reaction when I heard Gary say, *"I'm OK, pal"* that I had an hour earlier when I saw video of the explosion on the television in the breakroom at work: I broke out in tears.

One day later and I still can't explain why the incident struck me the way it did. Maybe it's because the Boston Marathon provided me with some of my fondest running memories. Maybe it's because I had many friends and club members run the Boston Marathon this year, some for the very first time. Maybe it's because I paced one of them to their Boston-qualifying race to get them into this event for their very first time. Maybe it's because I could have been running in the marathon; there was a time not too long ago when it was an annual ritual of mine. Maybe it's because if I had run this year's Boston Marathon, my finish time would have been very close to the moment the bombs exploded. Maybe it's because the Boston Marathon will never be the same.

The lasting image of this year's Boston Marathon is of a photograph I saw. It was the three-stripe Adidas logo (the long-time sponsor of the race) and the Boston Marathon unicorn logo on the sidewalk of Boylston Street...splattered with human blood.

Certainly, the Boston Marathon will never be the same.

THE BIG THREE

APRIL 17, 2013

During last week's Masters, the opening ceremony of golf's most illustrious weekend was perhaps the most replayed segment of the tournament on the *CBS* broadcast: golf's "Big Three," Arnold Palmer, Gary Player, and Jack Nicklaus, each hitting a ceremonial drive off of the first tee at Augusta National. For a person like me who grew up playing golf in the early 1970s, it brought back a lot of vivid and exciting memories of a time when a golf ball was hit off a tee with wooden clubs.

Tonight, my oldest running friends Al and Valerie joined me for a ceremonial run as part of a memorial tribute to this year's Boston Marathon. As it was for me, at one time the Boston Marathon was Christmas in April for both of them. In fact, the three of us made the trip to Boston together many times in a 10-year span starting in 1994 and we have the same number of Boston Marathon finishes: 12. At one time the three of us were referred to in running circles as the "Three Amigos," not only because our training philosophy was based on staying in marathon shape year-round (because you just never know when a marathon was going to break out), but also because we took it to the next level by running as many marathons as our busy schedules allowed. The three of us collectively have somewhere in the neighborhood of 450 marathons to our credit; many of them we ran together.

The evening produced a decent turnout for an event with little more than 24 hours advance notice. Al, Val, and I posed for a photo, the three of us side by side in the same formation we were photographed in almost 19 years ago to the day after we finished the 1994 Boston Marathon, the first of several we would travel to together. We, along with 60 or 70 others, then gathered for a group photo for the local newspaper, followed by a moment of silence to pray for the many lives impacted by Monday's atrocity. Then a simple command from the club president: *"Let's run 6.2 miles!"*

Al, Val, and I ran together as we had for many, many miles before, reminiscing about our favorite memories of the many trips to Boston and wondering if we had enough gas left in our tanks to qualify for the Boston Marathon one more time. Based on our individual efforts, finishing a simple 6.2 miles in the twilight of a warm April evening, we realized how much work we all have to do to find our way back to the starting line in Hopkinton any time soon.

But forgive me if I had images of Palmer, Player, and Nicklaus in my head as the three of us completed the 6.2-mile route which started and finished at the Peachtree City Library, a favorite running route of the local running club, the very same club of which I was president when the three of us started running together so very many years ago.

Getting old has its privileges, so I'll take that privilege and call Al, Val, and me the "Big Three." At least for tonight, even if it's only for one memorable 6.2-mile run.

There was a great post on Facebook last Monday not long after the senseless destruction along the finish line of the Boston Marathon: *If you're trying to defeat the human spirit, marathoners are the wrong group to target.*

I can't help but think it's in the cards for the Big Three to celebrate Christmas in April once more.

EIGHT IS ENOUGH

MAY 2013

Today I hosted the 11th edition of the Darkside 8-Hour Run, an annual springtime event where runners do exactly what the name of the event implies: run as far as they can in eight hours.

Ten years ago this month was the first installment of this event. In 2003, I decided to run at the local 400-meter rubberized track for eight continuous hours as I wanted to experiment with my hydration techniques in preparation for my upcoming 135-mile run across Death Valley (the Badwater Ultramarathon) two months later. I invited all my friends to join me. While many ran several laps and some several miles with me, no one opted to run the entire eight hours with me. So, by default I was the winner of the inaugural Darkside 8-Hour Run with 52.5 miles (the runner-up had 17).

In the years that followed the event has had its fair share of everything under the sun. It's been held on a 400-meter rubberized track and a .423-mile path around a pond. It has started at 8 a.m., 4 p.m., midnight, and once at 10:15 p.m., the latter in anticipation of a "sunrise finish" at 6:15 a.m. the following morning. It has subjected runners to temperatures in the low 70s as well as temperatures in the high 90s. There have been occasional encounters with wind and rain and one particularly frightening encounter with monsoon-like conditions with a little thunder and lightning thrown in for good measure, requiring a one-hour "timeout" until nature had restored order.

But this year's event, held on a 1.02-mile circular asphalt driveway in the beautiful environs of Bear Creek Farm in Moreland, Georgia (featuring a 7 a.m. start), knocked the "timeout" year out of the top spot with steady rains throughout the entire day and the occasional (and frequent) downpour, heavy winds, and unseasonably cold temperatures in the mid-40s. The wind chill made the conditions throughout the day resemble something you might encounter during February in Minnesota rather than May in Georgia. Some of the runners thought there was sleet at certain spots on the route. Two things I do know for certain: (1) I have never seen my breath before during the month of May in the 34 years I've lived in Georgia, and (2) I am so, so thankful to Hal and Linda, our hosts for the race, for opening their property to our group of 30. I also know (so I guess that makes three things I know for certain) that without the roaring fire Hal started in the fireplace in the outdoor pavilion serving as race headquarters, we may have encountered some serious cases of hypothermia with not only the runners but the volunteers as well.

Today reminded me of the 2009 Tallahassee Ultra Distance Classic (50 miles) when runners were subjected to steady temperatures in the high 30s throughout the day and even steadier heavy, heavy rains *all day long.* I went on to win the men's masters (ages 40 and over) championship that horrific December day, but in all honesty what I really won was the battle of attrition: There were only 7 finishers from a starting field of 27 runners.

The Darkside 8-Hour Run has a great history. Some runners compete for induction into the Oval of Honor that is reserved for men who run 48 miles or more and women who run 40 miles or more. Jeff Olive currently holds the men's event record with 56.68 miles; the women's record holder at the moment is Beth McCurdy with 50.34 miles. Joe Fejes, who currently holds the world record for the 72-hour run with 329 miles (he did it just over four months ago) is in the Oval of Honor with 52.03 miles (making this the only event I can claim to be one-up on Joe). Rico Dorsey, this year's 8-Hour champion, will be competing in the Badwater Ultramarathon a little over two months from now; perhaps he was using today's event for the same reason I did 10 years ago.

I started my day today as I do any other day when I direct a race. I woke up at 1:30 a.m., drank a couple cups of coffee, and went for an 8-mile run. On eight-hour race days in the past I usually managed to sneak in another 5 to 20 miles of running during the event.

Today, however, was a much different story. I kept waiting for a break in the weather to run a couple of laps but that break never came. My 8-mile run at 2:30 a.m. would be my only run of the day.

On this particular day, eight was enough.

FAREWELL TO AN OLD FRIEND

MAY 2013

A couple months ago, I read in the local newspaper that several schools in Fayette County would be closing soon. One of them was Brooks Elementary School, a quaint little school in a quaint little town not far from my home.

The school hosts a road race on the second Saturday in May every year in conjunction with their annual Brooks Day celebration. The race was founded in 1983, making today's race the 31st running of the event. I first ran the Brooks Day 10K in 1986 in a solid time of 37:44, good enough for 14th place. I returned the next year and moved up a few spots, finishing in 6th place. In 1989, I was given race number 1 as I had the fastest estimated time of all the race applicants: 37:30. As fate would have it I ran exactly 37:30, but several members of the Atlanta Track Club Men's Competitive Team competed, and I wound up in a disappointing 9th place. My best Brooks finish was in 1999 when I took 4th place. While I've never won at Brooks as my friend Bob Dalton has done many, many times (I might also add that today was Bob's 22nd consecutive Brooks 10K), I've always enjoyed running in the beautiful countryside of this quiet little town.

In 2006, I ran both the 5K and the 10K with one of my training partners, Paula (the 5K begins at 8:00 a.m. and the 10K at 8:30 a.m., so if you can finish the 5K in less than half an hour you have time to run the 10K). In a performance for the ages Paula was the first female finisher in *both* events; as for me I finished an overall 7th in the 5K and 22nd in the 10K, but I had a blast tagging along for the ride and seeing Paula win both races.

As I mentioned, Brooks Elementary will be closing its doors for the last time later this month. The closing of the school may also signal the end of the race, as the school's PTO has been the driving force behind the race for many years.

I ran the race today so I could pay my respects to the good people of Brooks Elementary School for all their hard work over the years. I have so many fond memories of the Brooks Day Race (now Brooks Beat) that you can't find in the majority of today's "big" (read: major sponsors!) races:

- Walking the halls of the school to use the restroom one last time before the race and seeing all the students' drawings and paintings proudly displayed on the bulletin boards.

- Heading over to the Brooks Day festivities after the race and watching the kids playing T-ball, while following the sweet aroma of fresh funnel cakes so I could replace the calories I had just burned off running.

- Attending the awards presentation and listening for the names of the runners I ran with every weekend as they were called up to the main stage to accept their awards.

- Receiving the simple-yet-oh-so-appropriate cotton T-shirt with the school's heritage proudly spelled out on the front and all the generous local sponsors listed on the back.

So here's to you, Brooks. You've had a good, long run. You should be proud of what you've done for running, for your community, and most important of all for your children.

As for me, I'm just proud you've given me the opportunity to support your race and run through your beautiful town these past 27 years.

YOU CAN CALL HIM AL

MAY 19, 2013

You may remember I met Al Barker on Thanksgiving Day, 1993. I had paced my friend and training partner Valerie in the Atlanta Marathon, where she had just qualified for the Boston Marathon for the very first time. Al congratulated Val, and the two of them made plans to run Boston in five months' time, since Al had already run a qualifying time as well. I, however, did not run a qualifying time. (They're based on a runner's age and gender, and the time Valerie and I ran was not fast enough for a 38-year-old male). So the two of them conspired to get me to run a Boston qualifier so I could join the party in April.

A little over two months later the three of us made a 24-hour round trip to Florida so I could bust a gut and run a Boston-qualifying time in the Tallahassee Marathon while Al and Valerie ran the same event at a leisurely, conversational pace to "show their support." Two months later the three of us ran the prestigious Boston Marathon, and as you already know, it wouldn't be the last time the three of us made the pilgrimage north for Patriot's Day weekend in Massachusetts.

Since 1993 Al and I have run together practically every weekend. For many, many years we ran our Sunday 20 (miler), only missing it on the occasion when one or both of us were out of town—in most cases to run a marathon. Now we meet every Saturday at Al's house at 5:30 a.m. for our regular 10-mile out-and-back run on the country roads of Fayetteville, Georgia. Today, 10 is the new 20 (a few years ago it was 15 is the new 20, so in a few more years it may change again).

I've chronicled our history together throughout my first five books, all of them about running. It's not uncommon for runners to show up at Darkside Running Club events and ask me to introduce them to Al, because they feel like they know him from the many stories I've told about him. I won't repeat any of them (in detail, anyway) here because they've been told in print before. (That, and I can always stand to sell a few more books.) But I will tell you Al turned 68 years old today, and he celebrated it by doing an amazing 81 push-ups in 60 seconds. Did I mention Al turned 68 today?

Al's legacy depends on whether you find the glass to be half empty or half full. Let's start with the half-full legacy:

Al is the only runner I know who has run a sub-five-minute mile, a sub-three-hour marathon, 100 marathons, and 100 miles in less than 24 hours. He is a licensed optometrist, an amazing artist, and a wonderful photographer. Cindy and I have three of his oil paintings hanging in our house as well as a framed 20-by-30 photograph Al took of local landmark Starr's Mill in our living room. Many of Al's friends have his paintings on display in their homes as well. He has also been a very good friend of mine for almost 20 years.

As for the half-empty legacy, let me just say that today he contributed to the legend of Al Barker. As he was painting in his North Carolina cabin, he (as he stated on Facebook) admitted to dipping his paintbrush in his cup of coffee instead of his can of paint by mistake. Beyond that tantalizing tidbit, you'll have to read about him in any of my five prior books (I could use the royalties!).

In a few days, he will make another contribution to the half-full legacy as he will be giving a mutual friend of ours a painting that will grace her family's home for many years to come.

Happy birthday, Al. May there be many, many more.

I'm just not ready to give up our Saturday runs any time soon.

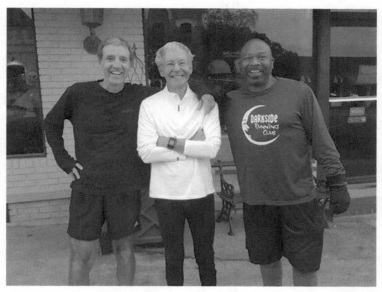

Scott, Al, and Antonio after a Christmas morning run through Senoia, Georgia

DFL

JUNE 2013

I like to finish what I started regardless of how much it hurts and how much I hate doing it.

School is a perfect example. I would have much rather been out riding my bicycle (elementary school years), going out on dates (high school years), or drinking beer (college years) than learning about the reproductive system of earthworms, the musings of Frank Kafka, or the gross national product of Indonesia. But I stuck it out—for a little over 17 years until I called it quits after earning a master's degree at the University of Florida.

The best example of finishing what I started is seen in my running.

In 1982, I attempted a 280-mile solo run across the state of Georgia. Beginning in Phenix City, Alabama, and heading east toward Savannah, Georgia, I pulled up lame after 159 miles on the morning of the fourth day. I hadn't anticipated the toll that running on the canter of the same side of the road would have on my knees. Ten years later I returned to the scene of the crime to rectify my first Did Not Finish (DNF) and completed the run across the widest part of the state of Georgia along Highway 280 (purely coincidental that the highway number and the total mileage of the run were one and the same!). This second attempt was successful for several reasons: (1) I alternated running on *both* sides of the highway to lessen the stress on my knees; (2) the run was conducted in support of a favorite charity of mine, and I didn't want to disappoint; and (3) I was absolutely intent, bound, and determined to finish what I started. Besides, I didn't want to return for a third time, which is exactly what I would have done had I not made it all the way to Savannah in 1992.

In 1988, I competed in my first 24-hour run. My goal before I began circling the 1.01-mile asphalt path around the water reservoir in downtown Atlanta was to complete 100 miles. When I completed my 100th mile (and 99th lap), I ran one additional lap for insurance (in case my lap counter missed a lap) and called it a day (night?) after running a little over 19.5 hours. I regretted not running those remaining 4.5 hours for a long time before vindicating myself and running the duration of a 24-hour run in Ohio in 2002, finishing with 129 miles and change…and sneaking in a masters (age 40 and above) National Championship along the way.

In 2004, I competed in the Western States Endurance Run, a trail run through the Sierra Nevada Mountains in California starting in Squaw Valley and finishing 100 miles away in Auburn. After running, walking, and crawling 62 miles I called it quits because quite frankly my knees were a wreck. The pounding they absorbed running up and down (mostly because of the down parts) the mountains had taken quite a toll, and although it was entirely possible for me to complete the final 38 miles in the 12 hours I had remaining (the race has a 30-hour time limit, and I had covered 62 miles in just over 18 hours), I wasn't convinced I wanted to do it on my hands and knees. So I cried "Uncle," only to return two years later to try again. The second time the conditions were treacherous and offered a little bit of everything: knee-deep snow, ankle-deep water puddles, and over 100-degree temperatures. Oh, and a series of 16 or 17 checkpoints along the course that had strict time limits: If you missed any of the checkpoint cutoffs, you were removed from the race. Somehow, someway, I managed to finish in front of all of them and in the spirit of full disclosure, until I reached the cutoff at mile 43 I was actually hoping to miss one of them and thus end my misery. From that point on, however, I wanted to finish the race if for no other reason because I knew I would not rest until I made it to the finish line of arguably the most prestigious ultramarathon in the United States. I was reaching checkpoints literally two or three minutes under the time cutoffs, the key word being "under." In many cases the runner(s) directly behind me were missing the time cutoffs; I could tell by their cries of anguish after they were informed they were not allowed to continue. When I reached the final checkpoint at 97 miles I had accumulated a 15-minute cushion; however, I was exhausted and was forced to walk 2.8 of the remaining 3 miles, breaking into a run only when I made my way onto the track at Placer High School in Auburn and running the remaining 0.2 miles to the finish line. I was the last runner to finish the race (only a little over half of the field finished—I told you the conditions were treacherous!). My official time was 30:16:58 (after reaching the final checkpoint a runner can take as much time as they need to make it to the finish line), and I was awarded the traditional last-place finisher's plaque and interviewed by the local news media. Not bad for a last-place finish, the key word being "finish."

In running, a last-place finish is affectionately known as DFL, or Dead F__ing Last (use your imagination).

However, in running DFL trumps DNF (Did Not Finish) that in turn trumps DNS (Did Not Start).

I like to finish what I start. Occasionally it may take a little longer than I would like, but eventually I'll get there.

WESTERN STATES

JUNE 2013

Seven (as well as nine) years ago today I was in Squaw Valley, totally out of my element. I was on the starting line of the Western States Endurance Run.

Some of you may not be familiar, so let me refer to the event's website to explain:

The Western States 100-Mile Endurance Run is the world's oldest and most prestigious 100-mile trail race.

Starting in Squaw Valley, California, near the site of the 1960 Winter Olympics and ending 100.2 miles later in Auburn, California, Western States, in the decades since its inception in 1974, has come to represent one of the ultimate endurance tests in the world.

The only word you need to focus on is "trail," because if you're natural running environment is asphalt (that being the case with me), running a race of any distance—let alone 100 miles—on trails can be quite the challenge.

Western States is not just any trail. For almost the first five miles of the race the route takes the runners directly up a mountain. Not just any mountain: the initial climb of 2,550 vertical feet up to Emigrant Pass at an elevation of 8,750 feet leaves you breathless and a with a sudden case of "sausage fingers," a phrase that is hard to explain but easy to understand when you see it in action (the extreme altitude and exertion causes your fingers to swell to the size of rather large sausage links—scary stuff if you're not used to it, which I'm not).

As you already know, my first attempt running Western States in 2004 was a dismal failure. Although I was well ahead of the pace required to complete the race within the 30-hour time limit, my knees had absorbed such a pounding from running up and down and up and down and up and up and up (and down) that I was forced to surrender after 62 miles. Ironically, from what I was led to believe by the veterans of the event, the heavy lifting was over once you reached the 62-mile mark. The last 38 miles were gravy.

Two years later I would return, only to discover for myself that those veterans had been lying to me.

At the very least the final 38 miles were just as difficult as the first 62. At least I believe they were; it was a little hard to tell for sure because I ran a great portion of them in the dark. At Western States, you're allowed to utilize a pacer (another runner—ideally fresh and rested who can run with you and make sure you don't do anything stupid like fall off the side of a mountain) after 55 miles if you reach that point after the sun goes down (which I did). Danielle did an outstanding job keeping me on pace, on course, and on track to finish under 30 hours. Western States has a series of checkpoints along the course that you must reach within a certain time limit; if you don't you are unceremoniously removed from the race. Although I was barely dodging bullets (hitting the checkpoints with only a minute or two to spare) throughout the night and into the morning, I was still in fact *dodging each and every bullet!* After 38 miles of watching over me, Danielle's problem with *her* foot forced her to turn the pacing duties over to Susan for the final seven miles. After reaching the 94-mile checkpoint in time, I ran my a** off for the next three miles and hit the 97-mile checkpoint with a 15-minute cushion. That was the good news.

The bad news: I was totally exhausted.

The good news: Once you reach the 97-mile checkpoint within the allotted time, you can take as much time as you want/like/need to get to the finish line.

The bad news: I did.

The good news: I still had enough gas in the tank to *run* the last 300 yards to the finish line banner on the high school track in Auburn and receive a rousing ovation for being the absolute last finisher of the race. My time? 30:16:58.

After having a finisher's medal placed around my neck, reporters from several local television stations interviewed me. Although I didn't attend the awards ceremony, a friend of mine did, and when I woke up from the nap I took in my hotel room literally minutes after my interviews, I found a framed print lying on my chest, the award given for my position in the race. Apparently finishing in last place at Western States is a pretty prestigious thing.

Knowing what I went through to get there, it damn well should be.

Just ask everyone who didn't make it.

INDEPENDENCE DAZE

JULY 4, 2013

It's the Fourth of July in Atlanta. For most people that means grilling out with family and friends, carving up a watermelon, and watching fireworks at the end of the day. However, for me that means getting up before the crack of dawn and heading to the north side of Atlanta to run in the largest 10-kilometer race in the country, the Peachtree Road Race.

I moved to Atlanta in June of 1979. One month later I ran my first Peachtree. Today I ran my 35th. In other words, I have not had the opportunity to sleep in on America's birthday since I've lived in Atlanta.

There have been a lot of changes in the event since 1979. I thought it might be interesting to do some comparisons between then (1979) and now (2013):

Then: There were 20,000 runners.
Now: There are 60,000 runners.

Then: Finish line was in Piedmont Park.
Now: Finish line is on 10th Avenue, parallel to Piedmont Park.

Then: Men's winner was Craig Virgin of the United States.
Now: Men's winner was Mosinet Geremew of Ethiopia. (Note: A Kenyan or an Ethiopian has won the men's division every year since 2000.)

Then: Women's winner was Heather Carmichael of New Zealand.
Now: Women's winner was Lineth Chepkurui of Kenya.

Then: Entry fee was $5 (if memory serves) and included a coupon for a free meal at Steak and Ale (that I used without fail each and every year it was offered).
Now: Entry fee is $35 and includes a coupon for a free waffle at Waffle House.

Then: I parked (for free) in the Lenox Square parking lot, about 100 yards from the starting line. A public bus returned me to my car after the race. For free.
Now: I park (for $10) in the parking lot about half a mile from the *finish* line. As I've done for the past six or seven years, I ran to the starting line before the race began. For free (as if anyone was going to pay me for it).

Then: I started about 30 yards behind the starting line.
Now: I started about 300 yards behind the starting line.*

---

* *Regarding my starting line position over the years:*

At one time I was able to qualify as a seeded runner at Peachtree. That meant I was assigned to the very first starting corral (with a three-digit race number) and was allowed to warm up on Peachtree Street with the Kenyans and the Ethiopians.

One year for the sake of journalistic investigation I started at the very back of the race (my race number was in the 90,000 range). It took me almost 90 minutes to GET TO THE STARTING LINE! My starting corral was so far back from the starting line that I warmed up by running north on Peachtree Street (instead of the southern direction of the race) and almost ended up in South Carolina.

This year my race number was in the 4,000s.

Then: I drank mostly water and a little Gatorade during the race.

Now: I drank mostly beer (OK, *only* beer) during the race. What can I say? Some of the Peachtree Street bars offer it for free; plus, it's always easy to get one from the generous fans enjoying their early morning brew along the course.

Then: I ran the Peachtree Road Race competitively, something I would do all the way through 2003. My primary (and perhaps only) goal was to run faster than 38:15. Anything slower than that would result in depression and a lot of what I referred to as punishment runs.

Now: I run the Peachtree Road Race in search of free beer, something I've done every year since 2004. What can I say? Since 2004 I've had three goals at Peachtree: (1) Finish. Success! (2) Beat my age in minutes, this year my target being 58 minutes as I'm 58 years old. I ran 50 minutes and change. Success! (3) Drink free beer. Success! No more post-Peachtree depression or punishment runs for me!

Then: The Peachtree T-shirt had the original, traditional large peach on the front.

Now: The Peachtree T-shirt featured yet another unattractive design chosen from an annual competition open to everyone with a pencil, paint brush, or crayon.

Then: I was younger and faster.

Now: I am older and slower.

Then: I thought to myself after the race, "I might run this again next year."

Now: I think to myself, "Just 15 more, and I'll make it to my goal of 50 consecutive Peachtrees."

Then: The race was hilly, hot, and humid.
Now: The race is hilly, hot, and humid. Some things in Atlanta never change.

Especially in July.

Postscript: There was added security at the race this year, a direct reflection of what transpired at the Boston Marathon a little over two months ago. Other than the fact there was a much more no-ticeable police presence this year, there didn't seem to be the least bit of apprehension among the runners. The Fourth of July is truly America's holiday.

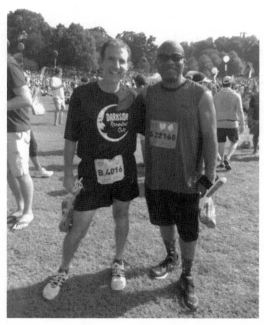

Scott and Antonio after Scott's 38th Peachtree and Antonio's first in Atlanta, Georgia

RAPTURE IN THE RAIN

JULY 2013

A couple days before the Peachtree Road Race the weather forecast called for a 100% chance of precipitation on race day. After having run this event each year since 1979—all in the heat and humidity of a typical summer day in Atlanta—I was excited by the prospect of running in the rain on the Fourth of July. In fact, when I got in my car race morning and headed to Atlanta, the first song I heard on the radio was Neil Sedaka's *Laughter in the Rain*. That song perfectly described how I was approaching the race because I was about to be transported back to the days when I was a little boy playing in the rain in the backyard of our home in Virginia Beach. I used to *love* playing in the rain. Still do, as a matter of fact.

So you can imagine how disappointed I was to run Peachtree for the 35th consecutive time without the slightest hint of rain. The only water I was exposed to was the water from several sprinklers along the course and a splash or two from a cup loosely held by another runner (at least I *think* it came from another runner, and I *think* it was water). Sure, it rained later in that afternoon (I'm fairly certain it has rained every single day for the past three weeks), but not one drop during the race. By the time it actually did rain later in the day, I was too exhausted (several beers will do that to a person, particularly if that person happens to be me) to get outside and enjoy the raindrops falling on my head (tip of the cap to B.J. Thomas).

I've had some fun in the rain in my time. Take a moment and get your head out of the gutter and I'll continue.

Thank you.

The fastest marathon I ever ran was in a steady rain, with a 20 mile per hour wind and a temperature holding steady at 38 degrees, rounding out a perfect day for me. I ran a personal best 2:48 marathon in those conditions on a cold winter day in Jacksonville, Florida, in January of 1988. The thing I'll remember most is that my teeth chattered uncontrollably for a good 60 minutes after I crossed the finish line—regardless of how much hot soup or hot coffee I consumed.

I ran in similar conditions in a half marathon in Toccoa, Georgia, in the winter of 1987. The only difference from that day in Jacksonville was the wind in Toccoa was blowing at a robust 45 miles per hour, greatly lowering the 38-degree temperature once the wind chill was factored in. To make matters worse, it felt like I was running into the wind the entire race, my singlet plastered to my chest for 83 minutes. I ran a good race, but trust me when I tell you I paid for it. The shower afterward let me know I had some major raw spots in two prominent areas on my chest that I made sure everyone in the men's locker room knew about by letting out the loudest, most blood-curdling scream uttered by a male in the history of mankind. That scenario would be repeated for many days to come. It was the first time Cindy ever suggested I give serious consideration to not running anymore.

Perhaps the most difficult and trying rainy day I ever ran in was in a 50-mile race in December 2009 at Wakulla Springs near Tallahassee, Florida. I have never run THAT LONG in such HORRIFIC CONDITIONS that NEVER CHANGED ONE IOTA THROUGHOUT THE COURSE OF THE DAY. When I say, "day," I'm referring to the entire 8 hours, 27 minutes, and 15 seconds it took me to finish the race. Forty-one degrees. Slight breeze, usually in my face (on a loop course, no less—*how is this even possible?*). TORRENTIAL DOWNPOUR! It rained ALL DAY LONG and came down in buckets. The entire time. I am not exaggerating. Twenty-seven runners started the race, and only seven of us courageous, unflappable, too-dumb-to-come-in-out-of-the-rain (pick one) diehards completed all 50 miles. I was pretty much miserable the entire day!

These three races were the absolute toughest (from the perspective of running in the rain) in a 35-year history encompassing almost 800 races.

But they all had a few things in common:

- Rain was prevalent throughout the entire race.

- The complementary wind and low temperature magnified the effect of the rain.

- When all was said and done, I had an absolute blast in all three races.

As I said earlier, I still love playing in the rain.

130 ON A SATURDAY MORNING

JULY 2013

As we do almost every Saturday morning at 5:30 a.m., Al and I went for our 10-mile run out in the country roads on the outskirts of Fayetteville, Georgia. Ordinarily our conversation is directed at solving the problems of the world and saving mankind; routine conversation, really for two eternal optimists and perpetual dreamers. But today we had more important issues to discuss: our weight, aging, and the 10-year anniversary of our trip to Death Valley for the Badwater Ultramarathon.

Weight: Al said after our run last Saturday in some really warm and exceptionally humid weather he weighed in at 132 pounds (normally he's in the mid-130s). I mentioned that I was as low as 144 pounds this past week (normally I'm in the mid- to high 140s; I know this because I weigh in on a freight scale at work every morning). I attributed the lower weight to the high humidity. Today it seemed the humidity was higher than a week ago, so we could only imagine what we might weigh after today's run.

Aging: Following our usual exchange of why we both wished we weren't working any longer, we talked about what we would prefer to spend our time doing—photography, painting, and traveling for Al; writing, reading, and watching *The Sopranos* from start to finish for me. (Fact: I have never seen an episode of the show, but have been told countless times I'll love it. Unfortunately, I do already know what happens in the final scene of the last episode.) Of course, both of us would still like to run, even if we're both having a little difficulty breathing today (humidity?) and running up the hills (age?). Al is 68, and I'm almost a decade his junior, but today there didn't seem to be any noticeable difference in how we were both faring: We were both struggling. Today I felt every bit as old as Al.

Badwater Anniversary: This year's Badwater Ultramarathon begins in two days. We discussed several of our friends who would be competing and reminisced about the 133-degree temperature readings everyone in Death Valley was subjected to a decade ago. As we have done every year since 2003, we joked that this year's Badwater competitors would probably see temperatures barely above 120 degrees, a veritable cold front compared to what we had to endure 10 years ago.

Admittedly today was not one of our better days. We walked quite a few of the uphills, and perhaps one or two of the downhills as well. We didn't solve world hunger or develop a strategy to boost the economy. We wondered if we were capable of running a single mile in the time that we used to *average* per mile in a marathon. (Sadly, very unlikely.)

But there's always next Saturday. Such is the curse—or the blessing, depending on how you look at it—of being the eternal optimist.

Toward the end of today's run, Al mentioned something around the eight-mile mark of "feeling 130." It just dawned on me that I don't know what he was referring to. His weight? His age? The temperature?

I've really got to learn to pay closer attention. Such is the curse—or the blessing, depending on how you look at it—of being the eternal dreamer.

TEN YEARS AFTER

AUGUST 2013

One of my favorite songs in the movie *Woodstock* is *I'm Going Home* by the group Ten Years After. Alvin Lee, the group's lead singer and guitarist passed away five months ago. On the day of his death I watched his performance at the greatest music festival of all time on DVD. Twice. This all has nothing to do with what today is about; I just wanted to call attention to how much I thought of the song.

But yesterday my wife and I did host a Ten Years After dinner party of sorts. We invited several of our close friends over to commemorate the 10-year anniversary of my adventure competing in the Badwater Ultramarathon during the summer of 2003.

After a book signing at the local Books-A-Million yesterday afternoon, Cindy and I hurried home to get ready for our guests who would start trickling in an hour or so later. Actually, Cindy did most of the actual getting ready while I completed all of the rigorous yet absolutely necessary making-sure-the-drinks-are-cold inspections. (In all fairness to me, I have to report that I tidied up the house earlier that day while Cindy worked at her store, took care of our grandson, and entertained her two brothers who were in town for the weekend. OK, so perhaps in perspective I really didn't do that much. But then again, I did have to run the automatic dishwasher since Cindy filled it up with a ton of pots and pans she dirtied preparing dinner and dessert for our party of 17.)

It was great seeing my running friends in street clothes. Having known most of them for 20 years or more, there have been very few occasions for me to see them in anything other than running shoes/shorts/shirts and sports bras. (I'm only referring to the women for that last one…if you don't take into account the time Al inadvertently strapped one on thinking it was his heart rate monitor, which if you think about it doesn't make Al wearing a cat sweater on his head one cold winter day believing it was his knit cap seem that bad after all.) I've got to admit: I've got some great-looking running friends. It's amazing what a difference it makes seeing a person relaxed, dressed up, and nursing an alcoholic beverage as opposed to seeing them on the brink of physical (and on occasion mental) exhaustion.

After an amazing dinner (compliments to the chef!), we all gathered in the living room to watch the 50-minute DVD of our 135-mile run, walk, and crawl across Death Valley just over 10 years ago. (Note: I officially competed in the event, while Paula and four others—Al, Eric, Gary, and my younger son Josh comprised the crew. Our success in completing Badwater, however, was truly a team effort.) Throughout the film I occasionally hit the pause button so the members of my support crew and I could provide commentary as to what the other guests were seeing on screen. Paula, my Crew Chief, mentioned she and fellow crew member Gary had a slight difference of opinion with my hydration plan. They also had a slight difference of opinion with the loading pattern of our team van. However, they both understood they were to protect me from all things negative so I could focus on running, and I have to admit they did a great job, since I had no knowledge of Paula and Gary's differences of opinion…or that they had lost my American Express card during the race…or ran out of ice at one critical point…or that Gary was in desperate need of medical attention around mile 70…or that my requested five-minute nap around mile 72 was actually only one-minute long (which would have had a drastic impact on me psychologically if I had known about it at the time).

Everyone seemed to enjoy the video, and I'll admit it brought back some great memories. Paula, Al, and Eric all said the same thing. We all wondered if we would ever find our way back to Death Valley again. Sandy, one of our guests, had just attempted running Badwater last month. A medical problem forced her to drop out of the race, but she has hopes that one day she will return to complete the 135 miles from Badwater, California, to the portals of Mount Whitney. I've known Sandy for a long time. I've seen her run a marathon in a pair of combat boots. She's completed numerous multi-day adventure races. She ran the Western States 100-Mile Endurance Run without the benefit of a pacer (I would have never finished Western States without one). She completed a 135-mile race in Brazil earlier this year. I know in my heart Sandy will return to Death Valley; in fact, I told her when she does I want to be a part of her crew.

That is, unless I'm healthy enough to try the race again myself.

THE LITTLE ENGINE THAT CAN

AUGUST 2013

This morning offered the first hint of fall: a dry 60 degrees. There's only one thing to do on an August morning as surprisingly wonderful as this: Put in a 10-mile run before heading off to work. And what better day to do it on than the day I'm going to see a neurosurgeon about my back problem, one who just might give me the same advice given to Paula several months ago: Stop running. So if I'm going to go out, I'm going to go out in a blaze of glory, 10 miles faster than I've run the distance in a couple of years. The run felt comfortable, but more importantly the run felt *familiar*. In fact, it almost felt fun again. Maybe there was hope for me after all. Let's see what the neurosurgeon says this afternoon.

Once I signed in at the Atlanta Brain and Spine Care, a nurse practitioner took my vitals and asked me a few questions about my back problem. I told her how I had experienced numerous and various pains below the waist for the past couple of years, but that the pains were now gone but the numbness in my right leg had gotten worse. I made sure to answer every yes or no question with "ma'am" at the end; I've made it a practice to do so whenever I'm in the room with someone who has the authority, power, or ability to stick me with a needle. I figure if that person is on the fence about whether or not I needed an injection, some blood drawn, or a friendly poke in the arm simply to prove I shouldn't be messing with them, my polite demeanor might steer them away from doing so.

Before long the neurosurgeon entered the room and immediately called me into the room across the hall to view my MRI with him. Two thoughts immediately came to mind: (1) He may as well be inviting me to interpret a page or two of hieroglyphics, because I have no proficiency whatsoever at interpreting MRIs, X-rays, or any other photographs of me taken on the *inside,* and (2) this can't possibly be good.

His very first sentence was (and I quote), "I see an MRI of a spine like this about once every six months" and then added he couldn't wait to tell others about it. In fact, he was a bit giddy when he said it. My very first thought was, "This must be the first time he's seen a problem like mine and now he will be able to write another article for a medical journal and add it to his collection of framed articles I noticed hanging on the wall in the first room I was in."

But then he went on to add several phrases that fueled the fire my grandson Krischan helped light several days ago when we went for a simple yet wonderful two-mile run together:

- *The spine of a 35-year old.* (Interestingly enough, I heard the *exact* same description of my spine from my orthopedic surgeon three years ago. I had my doubts back then, but now I have to believe there must be some truth in it.)

- *Pristine condition for a 58-year-old man.*

- Body has held up amazingly well for someone with 35 years of running under his belt.

- Genetically gifted.

That was some mighty flattering stuff for a first date.

He admitted that as much as he liked to fix people, he was absolutely *not* going to recommend surgery for me. As I had spent considerable time torturing myself on WebMD prior to my appointment, imagining what horrible fate might be in store for me, I'd be lying if I said I wasn't incredibly relieved to hear him say that.

He said he was a runner himself at one time and had run more marathons than he could remember, so he completely understood my frustration at not being able to run at 100%. I told him I stopped running marathons last year when I ran my 200th in Honolulu. We talked about running ultras, runners that both of us knew, races that both of us have run, the good old days when we were fairly fast, how once upon a time our common goal in races was to beat the fastest woman (not because we're chauvinists, but because there were some really fast women runners when we were both in our primes), and that we had the University of Florida as a common denominator (me as a student and him as a medical instructor at UF's Shands Teaching Hospital).

His recommended course of action came next. Yoga. Stretching.* Pilates. Physical therapy wouldn't hurt. I asked about massage and chiropractic treatments. He said he would try anything and

---

* *He asked me to touch my toes at one point during our conversation.*

 My feeble attempt—I barely could reach halfway down my shins—resulted in him pointing out my limited flexibility, a commonality in the runners he has treated.

 I told him the last time I touched my toes was after a hill workout in March of 1994.
 I wasn't kidding: I remember the day like it was yesterday, since it was also the only time I've ever touched my toes in my entire life.

everything, emphasizing yet again he would *not* recommend surgery. (Cue the dream sequence: I gave him the hugest man-hug of all time, lifted him up in the air, twirled him around in circles, and promised to have my next grandson named after him.)

So now it's up to me. I CAN get well again. I CAN run another marathon. I am the little engine that CAN.

I remember a slogan we had at JC Penney many, many years ago: *If it's to be, it's up to me.*
I want to run well again. I want to run another marathon.

There is a marathon in Fort Worth. Fort Worth, where my grandson Krischan lives. Could there be a better marathon to launch my comeback?

As fate would have it, this year's Fort Worth Marathon is on November 10, the same day as the Peachtree City 50/25K that I direct. Being an optimist, I interpret that as karma's way of saying it might be better to make my comeback at Fort Worth next year.

That way Krischan could be there to see me cross the finish line. There is nothing I would enjoy more than seeing his smiling face as his G-Pa drapes the finisher's medal around *his* neck. That way I could promise to be there when he finishes his first marathon and earns a medal of his own.

And if Karma opts to hang around for another 15 years or so, maybe I won't simply be waiting for Krischan at the finish line; I'll be running his first marathon with him.

But first things first: I must find a yoga class.

REACHING

AUGUST 2013

As has been the case for the past six or seven years, when the alarm went off this morning at 3:30 a.m., my first thought was "how am I going to make it through my run this morning?" followed by "I'll just take it easy today and run fewer miles and perhaps even walk some of it." As has *also* been the case for the past six or seven years, once I was 25 or 30 minutes into my run, I wanted to run well into the morning and thought "if only I didn't have to work today." That's how it's been with me lately and why I've had such a love/hate relationship with running pretty much every day since I turned 50. To make matters worse, I felt more tired than usual this morning, almost as if some part of me had been partying throughout the night while I was presumably asleep… as if there were some sort of celebration going on with my encouraging report from the neurosurgeon yesterday.

So how did today's run turn out? Just like every other run for the past six or seven years, but although the temperature was a few degrees warmer than yesterday and I ran a more challenging 10-mile route, I ran the same distance even faster than I did yesterday. To what do I attribute my fastest 10 miles in the last several years? One-part cooler temperature, one-part clean bill of health, and two-parts mind over matter. Dammit, numb right leg or not, I was going to run as hard as I could. I've blocked out a lot of pain in my life—a three-inch split in the bottom of my left foot at Western States incurred halfway into a 100-mile run in the mountains, running a hard marathon with my arm held against my chest due to a pulled muscle in my neck that caused me to pass out from pain after I crossed the finish line, countless dental procedures without benefit of anesthesia—so it shouldn't be too difficult to block something out that quite frankly doesn't really feel like anything.

After my run this morning I noticed a lot of comments about my "Little Engine that Can" story from yesterday that I posted on my blog (www.scottludwigrunsandwrites.blogspot.com). Many of them were congratulatory in nature while a couple promoted the benefits of yoga and stretching. Paula was mentioning a return engagement in Badwater. Valerie was planning our next Boston Marathon. If I didn't know better I would have thought I was cured, as in all better. But I wasn't better (not physically, anyway) as I still had to deal with my problems. I'm not out of the woods just yet, but I can definitely start to see the light.

"If it's to be, it's up to me." IF there was ever a time for mind over matter it was now. As I said, I'd like to run the Fort Worth Marathon. Sure, I'd like to run Boston one more time, especially after what happened there last April. Badwater I'm not so sure about, but I can tell you I missed being in Death Valley last month when two of my friends were there running in the race. Another 24-hour run would be my addition to the list, as at one time it was my favorite event. But back to square one, clearly labeled, "If it's to be, it's up to me."

Mentally my training began yesterday; today was the literal first step of my physical training. A long time ago I wrote an article about reaching for the stars. This time out I'll be happy to reach a single star. It might not be as fast or as pretty as it once was, but I know one thing for sure: It most definitely will be.

THE ACCIDENTAL MARATHONER

LABOR DAY 2013

I ran my 200th lifetime marathon last December 9 in Honolulu, Hawaii. At the time, it was going to be my last marathon for two reasons: (1) My body seemed to be literally falling apart, arguably from the wear and tear of running every day for over 34 years and (2) primarily because of the first reason, marathons were simply no longer fun. When I crossed the finish line in Kapiolani Park a short nine months ago I was more than ready to end my marathon career on a nice, round number: 200. "Unless I get my health back," I told Cindy at the time, "That will be my last marathon." Always a caveat, that's my motto.

Then one week ago today I was informed by a neurosurgeon that I was in much, much better shape than I thought possible, and life wasn't about being stopped by the wall but finding a way to get over it. Beyond that I had been having the desire—in spite of everything my body had been telling me—to run a really long distance again. If you recall I ran in a 12-hour event last March on a 1.03-mile loop course and intentionally stopped after 25 laps, or 25.75 miles, less than half a mile from the distance of a marathon. In my healthier, younger (aren't these really the same thing?) days I would do a run of that distance pretty much every week; in fact, many weeks I would do it more than once. Now I was only doing it once a *year?*

Then it dawned on me: I was letting the wall stop me, and the neurosurgeon saw no reason why it should. In other words, this was all on me.

So, after a week of the best running I've done in years I decided that today, Labor Day 2013, might be the day to try Marathon number 201 on for size. I was hosting my annual Darkside Labor Day Marathon and instead of running two or three of the more than 5-mile laps I decided I just might run all five laps. I had to wait for the last finisher anyway and figured it would be more enjoyable running than waiting around.

Despite experiencing the second occurrence of full-fledged vertigo in my entire life, I decided to give the marathon a shot. After all, the only other time in my life I had vertigo was the morning of the 2004 Boston Marathon, and by the time I started running the vertigo had dissipated, and I finished all 26.2 miles, thankfully on two legs. Sure, I was younger, faster, and certainly healthier nine years ago, but I couldn't dispute the incredible coincidence of experiencing two bouts of vertigo in my life, both on the morning of a marathon.

In Boston, it seemed that running allowed me to sweat out the vertigo; at least that's how I choose to remember it. Today I was hoping for an encore performance, because I'm here to tell you that setting everything up for the race, getting all the runners signed in, going over the instructions for the race, while spinning like a top was one of the hardest things I've ever done in my life. The worst? Unloading the tables and coolers from my truck, because bending down, over, or sideways was absolutely killing me, not to mention I was not truly bending down but actually contorting my body so I didn't have to bend, because bending made me downright nauseous. When I picked up one end of a large cooler (thanks for grabbing the other end, Sarah) containing three 20-pound bags of ice and lowered it to the ground—without ever bending, remember—I pulled a muscle in my side (but I didn't let Sarah know because I didn't want her to think I was a weenie and fortunately it was still dark so she couldn't see me wincing in sheer pain or the tears in my eyes).

So once the runners were on their way following my "Runner's, get set...GO" command, I followed in behind with the intention of running until my body started hurting. Incredibly that moment never came. At least not while I was running; that would come later in the afternoon, hours after I finished. But for those glorious twenty-six-point-two miles on this balmy, overcast day I was hearing the voice of the neurosurgeon telling me to find a way to get over the wall. Well, doc, I'm here to tell you, I did. Marathon number 201 is in the books. Nothing flashy in the way of my finishing time, but as I did nine years ago at Boston I crossed the finish line on two legs and more importantly *pain free*.

Cindy came out mid-morning to walk a lap. She was still hanging around the finish line when I completed my fifth lap and not once did she ask me how far I ran. I'm pretty sure she knew but the fact she didn't ask made me think if I didn't tell her I ran a marathon then it never happened. So I didn't. Tell her, that is. I *did* in fact run a marathon, and I actually feel kind of bad about it. Emotionally bad, that is; not physically bad. I broke a promise. I was not 100% healthy. Yet I ran a marathon, less than nine months after I said I wouldn't ever again.

Looking to put the blame for my indiscretion on anyone or anything other than me, a short list includes:

- The neurosurgeon's advice

- A week of pain-free running

- My personal desire to run long

Perhaps more than anyone or anything else, however, I must point in the direction of my friend Anne who told me a short time ago that ever since I stopped running marathons the world was spinning off its axis. That comment—along with its eerie correlation to my bout of vertigo—more than likely was karma's way of telling me to just do it.

SNAPP OUT OF IT

NOVEMBER 2013

I've done a lot of things in my life that, when I really stop and think about it, I realize I did them primarily because of how much fun it would be to write about them. For example, running 135 miles through Death Valley or vowing to touch my toes again after 20 years of barely reaching the lower part of my shins; you know, the spot where the shin curves and morphs into the top of my foot. What I did in October is one of those things: I ran a minimum of 10 miles every day of the month. "Double-digit days" is the name I gave them back in 1993 when I started running more and more of them each year.

Please understand I don't mean to boast when I mention running 10 or more miles every day in October (the truth of the matter is I ran 10 or more miles the last three days of September as well for a grand total of 34 consecutive days, but who's counting?) because 15 years ago it wasn't uncommon for me to run 10 or more miles virtually every day of the year, including *triple*-digit mileage on the weekends. Rather, I mention it because it is the perfect segue to introduce one of my friends to you: Craig Snapp of El Cajon, California.

Craig is a member of the United States Running Streak Association. To be a member you are required to run a minimum of one mile—under your own power, of course—each day for an entire calendar year. Craig, as well as his number one training partner Debbie, is the proud owner of a streak that began on April Fools' Day, 1998. I mention it because it is the perfect segue to tell you something else about Craig, something many of you may have a hard time comprehending, understanding, or even believing.

Up until July 15 of this year Craig had run a double-digit mileage for an amazing 1,870 days in a row. That would be a minimum of 10 miles each day for a period of 5 years and 15 days. And it's not like Craig took the easy route—as if there were such a thing as an easy route—by running *only* 10 miles each day just for the sake of reaching double digits. No, Craig took the difficult route, averaging a hefty 15.8 miles for each and every one of those 1,870 days!

I know what you're thinking right about now. The same thing I thought when Craig reached the one-year mark, then again when he hit the two-year mark, and a few more times after that: *Why?* Legend has it that Craig and Debbie were running with a mutual friend of ours and fellow streak runner, Prince Whatley. The three of them were discussing the statistics in one of my books when Craig mentioned he couldn't find one where he had me beat. (I guess he didn't notice his best marathon time was about six minutes faster than my best; shh, don't tell him!) Prince then asked him if he thought about trying a double-digit streak, and the rest is now history. The power of suggestion is a mighty, mighty thing.

Craig took a hiatus from his most extraordinary streak back in July when he was having a problem with his knee. He limited his run on July 15 to three miles, allowing his knee to be tweaked. Not to worry: Shortly thereafter Craig began another streak of running double-digit mileage each day.

His regular USRSA streak is well beyond the 15-year mark, and his lifetime mileage now checks in at slightly over 118,000 miles. Then there's this *other* streak Craig and Debbie have collaborated on that they began a couple of summers ago. Craig and Debbie have found money on the ground every day since July 14, 2011. But that's not something new to Craig. In his lifetime running career he has accumulated $1,790.93 simply by keeping his eyes on the road.

One more thing about Craig: He's a numbers guy like me. It shouldn't surprise you that Craig reports finding:

- 28,498 money finds (coins and bills combined)

- 143 bills found (currency analysis: 81 $1 bills, 26 $5 bills, seven $10 bills, 28 $20 bills, and one $100 bill!).

If you ask him, Craig can give you the breakdown of each and every coin and bill by denomination and date (for example, he has found 977 pennies from 2006 but only one penny from 1917). However, I should warn you, it's probably best not to ask because there are no guarantees when he might finish with his in-depth analysis of his unique version of collecting coins.

Several years ago, my friend Al ran every day for an entire year (as well as in November and December of the preceding year). On January 1 the following year, Al opted not to run, intentionally breaking his streak (Al can be a wise man at times, cat sweater be damned) and removing any doubt he might become one of the hundreds of active streakers in the United Sates.

Two days ago, I pulled an Al and intentionally ran less than 10 miles (9.5), thereby ending my consecutive day streak of running double-digit mileage. One month was more than enough and it felt...well, it felt like freedom, to be totally honest.

Two days ago, Craig ran 15 miles. The streak lives on.

He also found another 23 coins, keeping another streak alive: Twenty pennies, one nickel, one dime, and one quarter. Craig called it "the cycle." I can only imagine what you might be calling it.

NO PRESSURE

NOVEMBER 2013

I've been running now for 35 years. For the first 25 years I was hell-bent on running as fast as I could every time I heard the starter call out "Runners, take your mark…get set…*GO!*" When I first started racing I kept getting faster and faster, and as I did the desire to do well got stronger and stronger. Every race I ran was an opportunity to run faster or run farther—in many instances both—than the month before…the week before…the day before, in some cases.

Once I had been around the block a few times I started becoming increasingly familiar with the other runners in these races; specifically, the ones I would always set my sights on beating. When I first moved to Atlanta I raced quite a bit on the south side of town. That's where I met Hugh Toro, a runner the same age as me who would always finish a couple of steps ahead of me in the local 5K and 10K races. If it weren't for Hugh I would probably have three or four dozen "wins" to my credit from the early 80s, and the Salvation Army would have three or four dozen assorted trophies by now as I'm sure Cindy would have gotten tired of dusting them and asked (as in, insisted) me to get rid of them. Like she did with all my age group trophies a couple of years ago.

As I began racing more and more all around Atlanta I quickly identified the usual suspects, the runners I personally wanted to beat each and every time our paths crossed:

- "Duck Butt," a man a year or two older than me who always wore the same ugly striped shorts and waddled when he ran.

He was my nemesis in 5K and 10K races, and over the course of several years we probably broke even in head-to-head competition...although he never had any earthly idea I considered him to be my personal rival. How could he; we never spoke.

- "Knobby Legs," a man a year or two younger than me who had some mysterious lumps on the back of his calves and had the oddest "grinding" motion (his hips had a peculiar swivel to them as he ran). It kills me to say this, but he held the upper hand against me, but like Duck Butt he never knew how much losing to him bothered me...or that I even existed since I usually finished behind him.

- "Stinky Guy," a man the same age as me who was one of those genetically gifted runners who was competing at a different level than me. But I did beat him in a four-mile race once. Stinky Guy tried to get ahead of everyone at the crowded start of the race, so he ran up on the sidewalk, only to smash his head ('BOIIINGGG!') into a School Zone sign as he looked back to see where everyone was.

- Then there were the rest of the Usual Suspects I always wanted to finish in front of: The first woman (I'm not sexist, it's just that in my younger days I was always pretty competitive with the faster female runners in Atlanta), the heavy breathers (the ones who labor so much to breathe that it makes it difficult for *you* to breathe if you happen to be within earshot of them), and any runner who doesn't abide by the runner's code of proper decorum: Those pushing baby strollers, those wearing shorts with pockets and/or collared shirts, and those who have no concept of proper pacing (they'll run hard for half mile, walk to catch their breath, run hard for 1/3 mile, bend over and put their hands on their knees, run hard for…you get the idea).

The point is there was always someone I wanted to beat. It's not like beating them would offer me any fame, fortune, or recognition; rather, it was just something I felt I needed to do. Beyond beating the Duck Butts and the Knobby Legs of the world I was also competing against myself. I raced for many years with a predetermined time I wanted to run in any given race, and I always found myself doing everything in my power to achieve it.

For example, I would target a time goal of 38 minutes or less to run a 10K. If I ran faster than that I would go out for a celebratory run later in the day; if I ran slower than that I would go out for a punishment run. Either way I lost, because the additional run would account for another hour or so of my day. The pressure of competition works in mysterious ways.

Seven years ago, I ran 100 miles through the Sierra Nevada's. My body hasn't been the same since. The competitive days are over, and in a word, I find myself…relieved. My daily runs are more enjoyable and on the rare occasion I participate in a race, I simply enjoy the experience. The volunteers, the other runners, the fans, the scenery, the weather—*that* is what I'd been missing out on those first 25 years, and I'm more than happy to make up for it now.

I don't miss waking up race morning with butterflies in my stomach. I don't miss running so hard that it makes my stomach hurt. I don't miss having my legs turn into limp spaghetti. I don't miss feeling disappointed because I finished a couple of seconds behind Knobby Legs. I simply don't miss feeling the need to compete.

I've done my fair share of gut-busting runs, and I wouldn't trade them for anything. But these days I'm perfectly content with a simple run in the morning. No pressure, no expectations, and no disappointment; only the victory one finds in crossing the finish line at the end of each and every run.

That is the only win that matters these days. And I'm good with that.

PASSING THE TORCH

NOVEMBER 2013

I haven't run well in just over six years. While the yoga has been helping with my running the past couple of months, it's still nothing worth writing home about. Heck, it's not even worth writing about period, so forget I even mentioned it.

I met Ferit Toska, a graduate student from Turkey, at the University of Florida about a year after my running began its dramatic nosedive. In February of 2008 I was speaking at the exposition for the Five Point of Life Marathon in Gainesville, Florida. Ferit was in my rather small audience, and I could tell from the eye contact he maintained with me throughout my 40-minute presentation he had the desire to be a runner; one of the *best*. He spoke with me afterward and said he wanted to run the half-marathon the next day in 1:52, or as he put it, 5:20 per kilometer. I was going to be running the full marathon, but I said I would be glad to run the first 13.1 miles with him. In a pair of soccer shoes and with me by his side, Ferit ran his first half-marathon in 1:49. He hasn't looked back since.

Cindy and I have been friends with Ferit and his wife Gizem ever since. When we travel to Gainesville for a Gator football game or a race we spend the weekend with them, and when they come to Peachtree City for a race they spend the weekend with us. Two years ago this month they had their first child, a boy they named Derin. Today Cindy and I consider the three of them as family, and I trust they feel the same way about us.

Ferit and I run together every chance we get. When we do I offer suggestions to promote Ferit's talent at running farther and faster, while Ferit reciprocates by encouraging me to cut back on my mileage and allowing my body to heal. So far Ferit has been doing a much better job of listening than me, as he continues to amaze me with the speed and endurance he's been showing at such an early stage in his running career while I continue pounding my body with more mileage than I know I should.

A little more than one year ago Ferit and I went for a 10-mile run on a Saturday morning before a Florida Gator football game. I was still battling some leg issues at the time and failed to lift my right foot high enough to clear a slight rise in the sidewalk with only a mile left in our run. I hit the sidewalk with a perfect three-point landing, the three points being my right palm, my right elbow, and my right knee. All three were bleeding profusely as I lay there in the middle of the sidewalk. Ferit asked if I needed help. Getting to my feet, I said no while my body clearly was signaling for an ambulance. I looked up at Ferit and said, "I think it's time I passed you the torch," meaning it was now his time to be the better runner, the faster runner, the longer runner…and most certainly the *wiser* runner.

One month later Ferit won one of my favorite races, the Tallahassee Ultra Distance Classic 50-Miler with an outstanding time of 6:34:53. If you do the math you'll find he averaged less than eight minutes per mile…*for 50 miles!* I wasn't there to see it personally, but moments after Ferit won, the race director—a very good friend of mine—emailed me in amazement about Ferit's run. (Note: I told the race director before the race to watch out for Ferit.) I sent a note back to him saying pretty much what I said to Ferit four weeks earlier: It's about time for the torch to be passed.

This weekend the Toska's—Ferit, Gizem, and our "second grand-son" Derin—spent the weekend with us. Ferit was running in my event, the Peachtree City 50K. On race morning, I woke up early to get to the start of the race to get things set up. Before I left I put a copy of my book *Distance Memories* by the coffeemaker on the kitchen counter with a note:

Happy Birthday! You'll enjoy the chapter titled "Gainesville."
Be sure to read pages 237-239.
Today will be the official Passing of the Torch.

I wrote in those highlighted pages of four runners who have in-credibly bright futures in front of them. Ferit Toska is one of them.

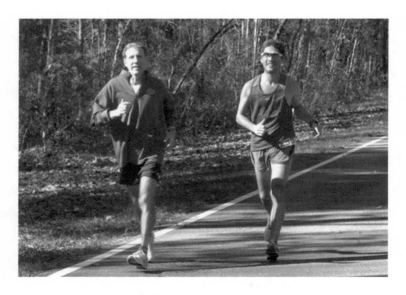

Scott and Ferit at Wakulla Springs, Florida

Ferit won the Peachtree City 50K today, running a spectacular race and finishing over 14 minutes in front of the second-place male.

The torch has now officially and unequivocally been passed. I trust Ferit will keep it burning for quite some time.

Footnote: Ferit won the Tallahassee Ultra Distance Classic 50-Miler the next two years as well.

PASSING THE BATON

NOVEMBER 2013

Yesterday was the 12th annual edition of the Peachtree City 50/25K road race. For all intents and purposes, it will also be the last.

The first race was held 11 years ago to celebrate the 50th birthday of my friend and fellow runner Paula May, one of the six original members of the Darkside Running Club. It was a very informal event in its inaugural year of 2002; in fact, it went by the moniker "Paula's Big Butt" at the time. Since then it's evolved into the largest of our club's annual events. In only its second year the race served as the United States Association of Track and Field's Georgia Ultra Marathon Championship, and in its third year as the USATF National 50K Road Championship. In fact, in the latter, winner Mike Dudley clocked the fastest 50K time in the country for the entirety of 2004 (3:05:34). For the 10th anniversary of the race (which also served as the 5th for the accompanying 25K), former Olympian Zola Budd Pieterse competed, setting a women's course record (1:47:06) for the 25K distance.

However, the event has failed to grow significantly over time and has yet to reach the published capacity of 150 runners in any of the 12 years of its existence. In fact, the number of runners has hovered around 100 for the past six or seven years, with a record high of 110 several years back.

What's disturbing is the race offers a great venue for both the runner venturing past the traditional 5K and 10K distances for the first time as well as the experienced long-distance runner seeking a personal best. The course is a winding, rolling 5.2-mile loop on the shaded asphalt golf cart paths of Peachtree City, and race day always seems to be blessed with veritably perfect weather conditions for runners, volunteers, and spectators alike. The race also offers something that's increasingly harder and harder to find these days: An affordable entry fee.

This year the entry fee was an all-time high of $50, and I'd be lying if I said it didn't bother me charging that amount. However, this year the recently restructured Peachtree City Recreation Department changed the rules a bit by adding a price tag to the formerly free-of-charge permit application of years past. The year before that they wanted more than just the release waiver signed by all the participants; the Recreation Department wanted an insurance policy as well. More and more financial obligations were tossed my way and with attendance not increasing over the years to offset these additional expenses, the entry fee needed to be raised.

Don't get me wrong: The $50 entry fee is still very reasonable in this day and age. It's not uncommon for a run-of-the-mill marathon to charge $100; big city marathons with big time sponsors may cost a runner upward of $150 or more. The New York City Marathon held earlier this month charged $266, and the Badwater Ultramarathon (135 miles through Death Valley) charged a whopping $995. So let me say this: $50 is indeed a very reasonable entry fee.

Yet the number of entrants for the Peachtree City 50/25K remains the same. It gets discouraging. Each year I hear those who run our event say how wonderful it is and that next year they're bringing some other runners with them. If that's the case, why aren't the numbers on the rise? And how do the races with those ridiculously high entry fees continue to sell out, year after year? (Don't even get me started about how the cities hosting these high-end marathons jack up hotel prices when the "captive audience" runners come to town.)

Al Barker and I founded the Darkside Running Club so we could give back to the running community. We're not in it to make a profit, but rather to use the profits to provide benefits to runners. Why else would we offer a one-time fee of $35 for a lifetime (family!) membership that includes a club patch, a quarterly newsletter, three free (!) marathons annually, and the opportunity to run in an annual club-sponsored event (Lake Hinson 24-Hour Run, Woodstock Running Festival) offering a stipend for participating? (The stipend for the Lake Hinson event in 2011 was $77 for each of the 13 club members who participated; in other words, they received their membership dues back plus an additional $42. Try finding another running club that does *that*.)

In 2011, I made a vow to myself: If the Peachtree City 50/25K did not reach the 150 entrant capacity it would be its final year. We fell about 50 runners short of our goal, and I was all set to give up the ghost, but several of the club members asked for one more year since so many runners had so many fond memories of the Peachtree City 50/25K and quite a few of them ran their first ultra there. In other words, they said all the right things.

So in 2012 I once again made a vow to myself: Either the race would reach capacity or a new race director would step forward or else it would be the last year for the event. Again, we fell 50 runners short...and no one stepped forward.

Against my better judgment I promised to do it one last time this year. I told the 300-plus members of the club and the 100 runners, this year would be the swan song for the Peachtree City 50/25K if it did not meet the criteria I set forth prior to last year's event. While many of the runners expressed both sadness that the event would be no more and appreciation for the 12 years of its existence, the event did not reach capacity nor did anyone step forward as the new race director. Sure, a couple of the club members expressed an interest (maybe more of a curiosity than an interest), but no one has taken the bull by the horns and said, *I'll do it!*

So on that note it's time to bid the Peachtree City 50/25K farewell. It's been a great 12 years, but as every runner who has ever crossed a finish line will tell you:

All good things must come to an end.

Footnote: The race would survive for another two years before it suffered the same fate as the Brooks Day Road Race.

STICKING WITH IT

NOVEMBER 29, 2013

I ran 10 miles this morning at 5:30 a.m. with my friend Al. It was 26 degrees when we started running and just as cold when we stopped, but nowhere near as cold as it was a dozen or so years ago when we ran 20 miles with a temperature that only amounted to a single digit.

But I've come to expect the running conditions this morning—and some a whole lot worse over the course of the past 35 years, because during this time I have run every single day; 12,784 consecutive days of running and 133,059 miles means I've averaged slightly more than 10.4 miles a day since a time when Jimmy Carter was President, *Dallas* debuted on national television, and Donna Summer's *MacArthur Park* (remember disco?) was the number one song in the nation.

Some might argue that my running is an obsession; others that it's an addiction. I'm not so sure either one is accurate, because I simply love to run. That's not to say I don't have an obsessive gene, however. I once did sit-ups every day for three years, with a daily minimum of 100 and some days with as many as 300. I once wrote a letter to someone close to me every day for 27 months, primarily for his emotional support but in all probability for mine as well. I've been doing my yoga regimen every day now for almost two months, but it's too early to say if this will develop into another obsession (addiction?). I once wrote a story a day for an entire year and published them in two books, totaling well over 1,000 pages.

I've had the pleasure of competing in almost 800 races, including 12 Boston Marathons, 27 Atlanta Marathons, and 35 consecutive Peachtree Road Races. In my younger (early 40s, an age I now consider "young") days at Peachtree I had the privilege of starting at the front of the race, literally rubbing elbows with the front-running Kenyans for several years (once the race started they always managed to leave me in their rear-view mirrors). One year recently I started at the very back of the 60,000-runner field to see what I had been missing out on. (Not much, I discovered; if you're not the lead dog the view never changes.) While I never won the Peachtree Road Race (non-runner to me more times than I care to remember: "You've run Peachtree 35 times, and you've *never won?*"), I did manage to win five races of varying distances, from 5 kilometers to 50 kilometers (3.1 miles and 31 miles, respectively) in my career. (Some might say I was versatile in being competitive at both short- and long-distance events; others might argue I didn't have any competition in the races I won. I know the truth, but I'm not saying.)

Running gave me the opportunity to run in some amazing places, such as Death Valley, the mountains of the Sierra Nevada's, Berlin, South Africa, Honolulu, and St. George, Utah. Running has also taken me—and Cindy (she always appreciated some of the destinations my race schedule took me)—to some amazing vacation spots: Boston, Washington DC, Tybee Island, Callaway Gardens, New York, Mobile, and Knoxville (she's been with me to Berlin, Honolulu, and St. George as well).

I've run as early (late?) as midnight and on one occasion as late as 11:30 p.m., barely squeezing in my minimum of three miles before the end of that particular day. I've run in the coldest of cold and the hottest of hot (133 degrees in Death Valley; case closed).

I've run in the wettest of wet (monsoon-variety rains) and the driest of dry (again, Death Valley; case closed). I've run in hail-storms, lightning storms, and windstorms. I've run when I was as healthy as a horse and when I was as sick as a dog. I've run when I was 24 years old and when I was 58 years old—and haven't missed a day in between. I've transitioned from newlywed to father to grandfather without missing a step along the way.

Tomorrow is another day. It will be November 30, 2013, for everyone else; for me it will be the first day of my 36th year of… Running. Every. Single. Day.

Have I mentioned I love to run?

ADIOS

DECEMBER 5, 2013

"Nana" was what my sister and I called my mom's mom, making her our grandmother on our mom's side of the family. Known as Thelma March Peifer to everyone else, she was always Nana to Hope and me. As my mom was an only child, we were her only grandchildren. Knowing what I know now about how much a grandchild means to a grandparent, I think back to the time I spent with her as a child and have a better and clearer understanding of why it felt so special.

Today would have been Nana's 107th birthday. She's been gone now for over 14 years, having passed away during the weekend of the 1999 Boston Marathon. My mom didn't tell me about Nana's death until I called her a few hours after crossing the finish line. It was literally a few seconds after I finished telling her I ran one of my better Boston Marathons while wearing the shoes Nana gave me for Christmas (a pair of running shoes made by adidas, known as the Adios). I loved how those shoes felt when I ran in them and loved even more the thought of Nana knowing they were something I would really enjoy and appreciate. I can tell you this: I never felt prouder wearing a pair of running shoes than when I was wearing the Adios. When you run with pride you tend to run well, as I did with my blue and white adidas Adios.

I ran in the Shamrock Marathon in Virginia Beach about a month prior to Boston. Although I was merely pacing a friend at Shamrock I still ran a good race; it goes without saying I was wearing my Adios. By that time Nana was now living with my parents since it was impossible for her to continue living on her own in Birdsboro, Pennsylvania—the small town she had lived in her entire life up until that point. The day after I finished running Shamrock I was getting ready to leave the house for the airport to fly home to Atlanta. I stopped in Nana's bedroom to say goodbye and tell her how much I appreciated her Christmas gift. While she didn't say anything aloud, her smile spoke volumes. Although I had no way of knowing it at the time, it would be the last time I would ever see her smile.

Now whenever I run in a pair of adidas, whenever someone speaks of the Boston Marathon, or whenever I'm with my grandson, I can't help but think of those special times with Nana. They all seem to bring a smile to my face, just like the one Nana always had for me.

Happy birthday, Nana.

2014

A CHANGE
OF DIRECTION

THE EMPEROR'S NEW SHOES

JANUARY 2014

I started 2014 with a resolution of doing 50 things I've never done before. My way of saying goodbye to my 50s since I would be turning 60 in December. Of all the things I knew prior to January 1 that I wanted to do for the first time this year, none caused me more anxiety, more apprehension, or more cause for deliberation than what I did today.

I'm making a special notation in my running log to mark the occasion: January 25, 2014: *I finally ran in my Hokas.*

You see, I've had my pair of size 10 Hoka One One's (that would be the official name of the shoes) in their original box in my closet since September.

September of 2012.

So you may be wondering why they're making their first appearance today.

What can I say? I like to live on the edge, and what better time to run in Hokas for the first time than 2014, my Year of Living Dangerously.

Let me back up for a moment. I've been having a variety of physical ailments and impairments ever since running, walking, and crawling 100 miles through some Godforsaken mountain range in California in the summer of 2006. (Fact 1: When it comes to running in the mountains, I am a fish out of water. Fact 2: If a fish remains out of water too long it will die. Fact 3: I believe you see my point.) Since that particular race I've been on a yet unfulfilled quest to find the perfect running shoe to absorb the punishment I subject my body to as I continue to run every single day.

A couple years ago I heard more and more runners commenting on how much they loved running in their Hokas. They were the new kid on the running shoe block, and everyone wanted to jump on the bandwagon. I began asking the runners I saw wearing Hokas what they thought of them, and without exception they were all huge fans. I saw more and more of them on the feet of runners of all shapes and sizes at various races. According to the favorable reviews I was reading and hearing, Hoka running shoes were living up to its company slogan: *Time to fly.*

So after giving it more thought than ever before about buying a pair of running shoes, I broke down and ordered a pair of Hokas online. The caveat was the cost: $169. Running shoe experts will tell you to expect 500 to 600 miles from a pair of running shoes. Doing the math, it appears it would be cheaper to drive a Hum-Vee 500 miles rather than run 500 miles in a pair of Hokas. At that price the One One's better do everything I dreamed of, if not more. At the very least I expected them to make me feel like I'm running along a path covered by a layer of cotton balls; best case scenario they will make me feel like I'm running on a cloud.

This morning, after spending the last 16 months in my closet, the Hokas found their way onto my feet for the very first time. I opened the shoebox—large enough to hold a toaster oven—and my One One's finally saw the light of day. *(That's a lie. It was 5:00 a.m. and even when my run was over the sun still hadn't made an appearance. Word of caution: I'm prone to lie at the drop of a hat.)*

"What an odd creature," I thought to myself. *(Actually, I said it out loud and our orange tabby Moe, who was sleeping in the chair I was sitting on the edge of to put on the Hokas, thought I was talking to him. I already told you I'm prone to lie at the drop of a hat; you can't say you weren't warned.)*

The white pair of Hokas sported HUGE heels that brought back memories of the white platform shoes I wore to my senior prom some four decades ago. There was an extra pair of shoelaces in the box, but for the life of me I don't know why because the shoes featured an intricate lacing system where the laces are threaded through a plastic gizmo that gives way to a leather whatchamacallit, and I couldn't see how the shoelaces could be removed since they actually formed one big loop with no loose ends. (There wasn't an instruction manual in the shoebox; by all rights there should have been.) Through a couple minutes of trial and error, I did manage to figure out how to tighten the shoelaces (it involved separating the blue and the gray halves of the plastic gizmo and pushing them back together once the laces felt snug).

At 5:30 Al and I headed out for our regular Saturday morning run. It was 16 degrees with a wind chill bringing the temperature down into single digits. I took my first couple of steps...and I can most definitely assure you I was not running on clouds. Not even a path covered in cotton balls. I remembered one of the runners I asked about Hokas telling me it took three or four runs until you could truly appreciate their performance. Three miles into my run I heard the familiar *clap* as my right foot struck the asphalt. "When will it be my Time to Fly?" I thought to myself. *(Again, I'm lying. I actually directed this question to Al, who had no earthly idea what I was talking about.)*

We interrupt this message for a brief public service announcement.
If you're running in expensive running shoes and stop on the side of the road to answer nature's call on a dark, cold, and very windy morning it is highly advisable to do so with your back to the wind. We now return to our regularly scheduled message.

So after my first 10 miles running in a pair of Hokas I'm disillusioned, disappointed, and just a little bit disgusted. Not as disillusioned, disappointed, or disgusted as when I ran in a pair of Sketcher Go Runs *(Can you say goodbye shins?)* for the first time, but pretty darn close.

Sure, I'll give them a few more tries in the next few weeks; after all I did invest $169 in them. But for now, I have to go.

It's Time to Cry.

Postscript: I wear my Hokas regularly, just not to run in because that would be crazy. Not $169-for-a-pair-of-running-shoes crazy, but close.

DRIVE BYGONES

MARCH 2014

As I do most of my early morning runs on the "deep south" side of Atlanta, every blue moon or so I find myself the center of amusement for one of the locals. For the sake of this story, I'll refer to the local as a Foxworthy.

Now that that's out of the way, here's what happened during this morning's blue moon. I was running my usual weekday 9-mile route when a truck with studded rubber tires almost three feet in diameter came barreling by at roughly twice the legal speed limit. But what the hell: It was barely 4:30 in the morning along a deserted country road, and the only lights visible were the two headlights on the truck and the tiny beam of light emitting from my flashlight. So apparently the Foxworthy driving the truck thought he would have some fun and veer toward me, forcing me onto the shoulder of the road.

What a jerk.

Only this Foxworthy wanted to double his pleasure. I saw him make a U-turn up ahead and head back toward me, ultimately forcing me onto the shoulder of the road a second time.

What an asshole.

I looked back, and you'll never guess what happened next. Yep, another U-turn. I gave him the benefit of the doubt and thought he needed to resume traveling in the direction he was traveling in originally. Although that might be part of the reason for the second U-turn, the rest of the reason is that he wanted to buzz me a third time, only this time his side mirror clipped me on the shoulder as he sped by.

What a Foxworthy.

Yes, three drive-byes qualify you as a bona fide Foxworthy in my book. That being said, here are a few things for you to ponder (think about—come on son: *Concentrate!*) while you're still a free man. I want you to know the differences between you and me, other than the one you already know: That I'm just a normal guy, and *YOU'RE A FREAKIN' MENACE!*

- I always brush off people like you because I know deep down you're simply jealous; jealous of someone trying to lead a healthy, active lifestyle while yours consists of NASCAR, chewing tobacco, and PBR. Let me clue you in, Foxworthy: You and I have LOTS of differences besides our lifestyles of choice.

- If I'm ever driving along the highway and my car craps out, as long as I'm within a couple hundred miles of civilization I'll be fine, because I could run there if I had to. You on the other hand will be stranded on the side of the road cooking up some roadkill barbecue on an open fire. (Armadillo on the half shell: They're not just a myth!)

- Over 40 years later I'm still at the same weight I was in high school. You were probably voted "most likely to become a dirigible" (look it up) by your senior class and from what I saw when you buzzed by me (no less than three times, Fatty Mc-Fatt), nothing seems to have changed.

- My resting pulse is around 50 beats per minute. I imagine yours is about twice that. I expect to live to be at least 90. How long will *you* live? Well, first of all don't multiply by two because your heart beats twice as fast as mine: You have to divide by two. (You *do* know how to divide, right?)

- My mode of transportation of choice is a pair of running shoes with one-inch rubber soles, while yours is a rather loud truck coated in mud and sporting 36-inch rubber tires...with about a case-and-a-half of empty beer cans in the back, from what I saw.

- My favorite exercise is running and while endurance is my strong suit, I doubt I could keep up with you doing your favorite exercise: 12-ounce curl repeats.

- My drink of choice after exercising is water. Your drink of choice during exercise is Pabst Blue Ribbon beer, meaning basically we're drinking the same thing so just you never mind.

- I make one or two trips annually to Atlanta, one to run the Peachtree Road Race and if there is another it's for a Florida Gator alumni function. If you make it to the ATL it's either because you've got a hankerin' for a Varsity or have to appear in a Fulton County courtroom for reckless driving.

If you ever do wind up in that courtroom—and I have every reason to believe that one day you will—you'd best pray I won't be sitting on your jury.

LONG WAY TO RUN

MAY 2014

Let's pretend a smooth asphalt road completely encircles the earth and follows the exact path of the equator. Now imagine my home in Senoia, Georgia, is located on that road *(it's not, but we're pretending, remember?).*

Now pretend I left my house for a run heading east, and I ran every mile I've ever run in my life all at once without stopping.

If all these things were true, then I would have been running through Jhang, Pakistan, this year on the last day of May.

Actually, if I never strayed from that imaginary path on the equator I would have been running through Jhang for the *sixth* time, as that was the day I ran my 135,000th lifetime mile.

As you may have already gathered I have kept pretty diligent records of my running for the past 35-plus years. My running logs have at least one entry every single day since November 30, 1978. The last day I failed to run—November 29, 1978—was due to an unfortunate problem with my stomach caused by something I inflicted on myself the day before. It could have been one of two things: (1) running 13 miles to win a bet with my college professor who knew the longest distance I ever ran was only eight miles, or (2) drinking a couple of celebratory pitchers of beer afterward, complements of my college professor paying off his lost wager. Now that I think about it, it was probably a little bit of both.

I've been a slave to numbers for as long as I can remember. I have always set mileage goals for myself: weekly, monthly, and yearly. In my prime if I set a goal of running 90 miles in a week, I would load up on the front end of the week to ensure that by the time the week was drawing to a close I would be assured of reaching my target. Inevitably this led to weeks of 100 or more miles because I would usually finish the week the same way it started: with high mileage. *(You can imagine the results when this philosophy is extended into months and years of running. That being said, 135,000 miles in 35 years should really come as no surprise.)*

As for being a slave to numbers, I have historically tried to tie in milestone mileage plateaus with something of significance in my running career. For instance, I reached 100,000 lifetime miles as I crossed the finish line of the 2005 Atlanta Marathon (one of my favorite races) and 125,000 miles on the 50-yard line of Florida Field in 2011 amid a welcoming entourage of my wife, the University of Florida cheerleaders, and what-Gator-celebration-would-be-without school mascots Albert and Alberta Alligator.

So I meticulously planned my week leading up to the culmination of running my 135,000th mile as I wanted it to be at the exact same spot where one week earlier Al, Amanda, and I found six abandoned kittens on the side of the road. It required a 20-mile run on Monday and a total of 36 miles the rest of the week, but it was well worth the effort. When Al, Amanda, and I reached the 9-mile mark of our 10-mile Saturday morning run, we stopped to let the moment soak in. One hundred and thirty-five thousand miles. The adoption of all six kittens less than a week ago. Another exhilarating, never-taken-for-granted run in the country. Good health. Camaraderie. Physical fitness. Friendship. The simplicity and purity of running.

The moment was special for a lot of reasons. It made me think of all the other special moments in my life, all of which I could affix a number to if I had the urge *(that number being my lifetime running mileage at that point in time):*

• The day Cindy and I moved from Florida to Georgia.

• The births of both of our sons.

• The deaths of Cindy's parents.

• The deaths of my parents.

• The birth of our grandson.

• The day we moved into our new house in Peachtree City.

• The days both of our sons graduated from high school and, for one of them, college.

• The day I said goodbye to the company I was with for 24 years.

• The day I said hello to the company I have been with ever since.

But assigning a number to these moments would be the wrong thing to do. You can't put a number, *any* number—whether it be mileage, value, or importance on a scale of 1 to 10—on the moments that define your life.

With that thought in mind I'm going to try my very best to quit placing numerical goals on myself. Lord knows I've tried cutting back on my mileage over the years, but I'll be the first to tell you the success has been negligible. If whether or not I've been successful at cutting back was up for debate, a novice debater might argue I have indeed been running fewer miles the past couple of years and therefore have successfully cut back. However, a veteran debater might concede I'm running fewer miles but that I'm still spending as much time on the roads since I'm running considerably slower than in years past and therefore have not technically cut back.

However, a *master* debater could bring the whole matter to an abrupt close by pointing out the obvious: Successfully cutting back requires less mileage AND less time spent running. *(Note: There is no such thing as a master debater. I just wanted to use it in print to see if it was as much fun reading it as it was hearing it said out loud. Footnote to note: It's not.)*

So today I vow to quit placing mileage goals on myself. I don't need the stress, the pressure, or the demand of running X miles each week, each month, or each year.

As long as I can run my 150,000th lifetime mile by the time I turn 65…

Postscript: The evening of May 31 Cindy and I attended a Collective Soul concert. The encore consisted of two songs: *Shine* followed by the finale *Run*. You may be familiar with the last line of the song, which is repeated several times before the song comes to an end:

Have I got a long way to run?

Karma can be a bitch. Or perhaps my ally. Sometimes it's hard to tell.

It's up for debate.

Postscript: Before the end of the year I passed 137,000 lifetime miles. I also passed 60 lifetime years. It made me wonder if 150,000 miles by age 65 was still realistic. It also made me wonder why I keep setting numerical goals that don't matter to anyone in the world but me. Old habits die hard.

BE LIKE MEAN JOE GREENE

JULY 4, 2014

I moved to the Atlanta area in 1979. In over 35 years the latest I ever slept in on the Fourth of July was that very first year: I slept until 5:00 a.m. so I could make it to the north side of Atlanta from my home in Rex for the start of the Peachtree Road Race, a 10-kilometer run through the heart of Atlanta. Back then the race had a field of less than 10,000 runners, and it wasn't hard to find a parking place in Lenox Square, a mere 60-second walk to the starting line on Peachtree Street.

This morning the routine was a little different. I woke up to a 3:45 alarm so I could drink a couple cups of coffee to get the cobwebs out and loosen up (both inside and out) before getting in the car at 5:00 and heading north on I-85. As has been my custom for the past several years, I took the exit that would take me to Piedmont Park—the coveted finish line where I would park the car and run to the starting line (to loosen up even *more* and yes, both inside and out). This year the congestion—even at 5:45 in the morning—was a little too much for my liking. There were a lot more detours than normal on the way to the parking lot, compounded by a policeman at every intersection. On one side street there was a policeman in a bright yellow vest spinning out of control, gesticulating wildly with his arms and shining his flashlight every which way that distracted me so much I drove straight through a stop sign. It was darn nice of him to point out my little indiscretion:

Officer Cuisinart: *"Did you see that stop sign you just went through?"*

Me (out loud): *"I was so focused on watching you giving me hand signals that I totally missed it. I'm sorry."* (My thought balloon, AKA the unfiltered version: *"Apparently not, Einstein."*)

Officer Cuisinart: *"Get out of my sight."*

By 6 a.m. I had the car safely parked about a half-mile from the finish line and began my five-mile warm-up run to the start. As I ran I thought about the days of Peachtrees past:

* The first one 35 years ago (only my fourth 10K ever and my first one in the state of Georgia) that I ran in 42:03. *(OK, I didn't really remember the time; I had to look it up. As I said, it was 35 years ago.)* Back then the finish was in the heart of Piedmont Park, and the common misperception for runners back then was that once they were inside the park it was time to sprint to the finish—even though there was still more than a mile remaining (a bit too long for a sprint, and yes, I made that mistake more than once).

* Consistent 37- and 38-minute finishes when I was in my 30s and holding steady in the 38-minute window into my 40s and earning a spot on the Atlanta Track Club Men's Masters (for runners 40 years and older) Competitive Team for a decade. I'll never forget the days of being in the seeded corral at the start and rubbing elbows with the human rockets from Kenya and all the other countries where the children wear T-shirts with "Oh, so you run a mile in under five minutes: How cute!" printed on them. While I had no legitimate business being in the seeded corral (it was easier for a masters runner to qualify for the seeded corral than it was for runners 39 and younger; after all age has *some* privileges), I really enjoyed having

volunteers bringing *me* water and wet towels as I stood on Peachtree Street waiting for the race to start.

- 1996, that magical year when it was 63 degrees at the start of the race (it's not unusual for it to be in the mid-70s with 105%—*no, not a misprint*—humidity for the 7:30 a.m. start), and I ran my Peachtree best: 36:56.

- 2004, the year the wheels fell off. I ran Peachtree a mere seven days after putting my legs through 18 hours of severe torture, punishment, and anguish running, walking, and crawling the first 62 miles of the Western States Endurance Run and convincing the medical staff it wasn't a good idea to amputate my right leg like they wanted to do. I ran Peachtree in a (then) personal worst 45:44 and realized on that day my wheels were indeed starting to fall off. Hmmm…maybe that medical staff had the right idea after all.

- 2005, the year Peachtree turned into a 'beer run.' My goal was to drink as many free beers as I could beg, borrow and/or steal along Peachtree Street. I consumed a 'personal best' of five beers before I reached the finish line. (In the 1990's I rode a bus to Peachtree with the local running club, and after the race everyone hung out in Piedmont Park until all of the members had finished. Back then I was drinking five beers just to rehydrate.)

- 2007, the year Susan Lance and I started at the very back of the race just to see what it was like. How was it? Let's just say it won't happen again. However, I will tell you we didn't cross the starting line until 9 a.m. (the official race begins at 7:30) and that our official (run) time was just a couple of seconds more than an hour…and that with all the darting and weaving

Susan and I had to do to maneuver around slower runners we probably ran a little over eight miles.

Back to today's race:

Whatever changes for the worse there were at the finish area (surely you haven't forgotten Officer Cuisinart), there were noticeable changes for the better at the starting area. There were no lines at the porta-johns (unheard of, even back in the days when Peachtree featured "the world's longest urinal"—a metal contraption about 50 yards long that allowed 100 or more runners the option of no waiting if all they needed to do was number 1). The walk to the starting corral was a breeze (compared to the past couple of years when that same walk was akin to being in the crowd outside of Wal-Mart when they open their doors on Black Friday). Even the volunteers seemed more pleasant and accommodating than usual, although it's entirely possible the volunteers have always been that way, but I noticed it this year because on the way to the start I saw a lot of runners I've known for a very long time and for the most part they looked a lot older than they used to; gee, I wonder what happened to *them?!*

As I waited for the race to start the announcer mentioned that Meb Keflezighi, this year's Boston Marathon winner, was at the back of the pack with the intention of passing something like half of the runners in the field for a fundraiser. I couldn't help but think Susan Lance and I did the exact same thing seven years ago, except that no one donated any money to charity for us to do it. We just did it *because.*

Once the starter said "go" almost two minutes passed before I actually crossed the starting line. I started out at a conservative pace, a pace that allowed me to notice free beer on my left from a Mexican restaurant about one mile into the race and two miles later free beer from a local tavern on my right. As I wanted to get a "Time Group A" seeding next year (requiring a finish of less than 48 minutes), I couldn't afford the time to belly up to the bar as I had done during my beer-run days.

As I made my way up Heartbreak Hill (about three miles into the run) I noticed the medical offices of the neurosurgeon who recommended I take up yoga as a way of curing the ills of Western States in my right leg. When I saw him 10 months ago he asked me to touch my toes. Laughing, I barely touched the middle of my shins. Today I can touch the back of my middle knuckle to the floor. In about three more miles I'll have a gauge to see if the yoga is helping my running. (Last year's Peachtree time? 50:24. Be sure to make a mental note: You'll need this later.)

Heading up the second hill leading to Colony Square—and in my opinion the more difficult of the two—I noticed two healthy looking men in their 20s stopping to walk and catch their breath. I couldn't help but feel proud of myself for keeping the same pace I had been running for four-and-a-half miles...when a young boy who couldn't have been more than 12 years old pulled up alongside me and asked me how far we still had to run. "About a mile-and-a-half," I told him. Well, actually all he heard was "about a mile" because he was 50 yards in front of me before I could get the words out of my mouth.

As I made the final left-hand turn to the final downhill leading to the finish line I felt good about my chances of finishing in less than 48 minutes. If I didn't trip over any speed bumps, street reflectors, or discarded beer cans I should make it with a few seconds to spare.

Thirty-eight. That's the number of seconds I had to spare. I crossed the finish line with 47:22 (actually 47:21:89) showing on my chronograph. It's official: I'll be in Time Group A when I line up for my 37th Peachtree Road Race, my first at the age of 60. (Note: The standards for sub-seeded times haven't changed. In other words, for me to rub elbows with the Kenyans ever again I have to meet the same standards set forth for a 40-year-old. Age has lost some of its privilege at Peachtree, but then again I *do* get a 5% discount on my groceries on Wednesdays. Also, the yoga appears to be working.)

Now for the moment I've been waiting for: My "Mean Joe Greene" moment. For those of you who don't remember (or never knew to begin with) there was a famous commercial for a certain carbonated beverage (that happens to be made in Atlanta) starring Mean Joe Greene, a player on the talented Pittsburgh Steeler team of the 1970s. After a game, a young boy—about the same age as the boy who dusted me on the Colony Square hill—handed an obviously exhausted Greene his bottle of soda on his way to the locker room. Greene gulped it down and started to walk away, only to turn around and say "hey, kid, catch" while tossing the young boy his jersey. The young boy—obviously—is overjoyed (*"Hey, thanks, Mean Joe!"*).

So after the race I picked up my Peachtree T-shirt (coveted in certain circles) and scoured the crowd lining the wire fence around Piedmont Park for just the right boy for my Mean Joe Greene scenario to play out. I walked a couple hundred yards and found my intended target: A boy of about 10 or 11 standing between his mom and dad with his eyes as wide as the coaster my beer is resting on at the moment. Perfect: His mom and dad aren't running so he won't be getting a Peachtree T-Shirt from them; he appeared to be excited about seeing all the runners who have just run in *the* Peachtree Road Race; and in all honesty looked a lot like what I imagine my grandson will look like in another five or six years. I smiled at the boy, tossed him my shirt, and said "hey, kid, catch" albeit not in the same deep, raspy voice of Mean Joe Greene. I walked a few steps, smiling at myself at the possibility of making someone's day when I heard someone run up behind me and grab my left arm.

"Hey mister, this isn't my size. Have you got one in a small?"

THIS 1812 WAS NO WAR

SEPTEMBER 2014

I don't know who was more excited this morning, my five-and-a-half-year-old grandson or his 59-year-old G-Pa. But I do know this: We both had the time of our lives.

I've had the pleasure of running with Krischan pretty much since the day he learned to walk. The boy loves to run, and I couldn't be happier. Or prouder, seeing as he wants to run just like G-Pa. In fact Krischan reminded me of my son, his Uncle Josh, when he first started running a couple of decades ago. It's been quite a spell between generations, but after today I can honestly say it's been worth the wait.

You see, this morning Krischan ran his first official race, and I had the pleasure of being there with him, every hop, step, and detour-to-pick-up-miscellaneous-odds- and-ends (baseball, pine cone, dead cicada) along the shady, hilly one-mile route near Spalding Regional Hospital in Griffin, Georgia.

After a busy afternoon and evening hunting invisible space alien babies in the woods behind the house, finding a jawbone that instantly transformed us into "scientists" (the "fossil" was later identified by a Facebook friend as that of a deer), and baking our requisite Friday night batch of peanut butter cookies, I woke up this morning at 3:45 to get in my 10-mile run with my friend Al...while Krischan slept in until 7:30 (our race was at 9:00). Of course, no five-and-a-half-year-old boy sleeps in until 7:30; rather he was woken up early on this Saturday morning by his Yia-Yia (my wife Cindy) to get ready for his racing debut. As you can imagine it wasn't pretty, but after he put on his shorts, shirt, and running shoes, he couldn't wait to get to the starting line.

"How much farther?" I heard more than once as we made the 30-minute drive to Griffin. When we pulled into the parking lot his eyes were as wide as the finishing medal he hoped to have draped around his neck once he crossed his first finish line. I didn't have the heart to tell him there probably wouldn't be a medal for the race (there was an accompanying 5K race—the big event; the one-mile was merely the accompanying fun-run), but if there wasn't he could choose one of mine when we got back to the house. (He's always admired my medal collection, and one day it is certain to be his.)

We picked up Krischan's race packet, and he instantly asked me to pin his race number to the front of his shirt. The number almost covered his entire stomach, but that didn't matter to him. He was now an official runner. We walked back to the car to drop off his packet, and although I had asked him several times just moments earlier if he needed to use the restroom while we were near the hospital, and he said no every time, once we were in the parking lot—with neither a restroom nor porta-potty anywhere in site—he had to go. *Now!* He ran to a tree, dropped his shorts to his ankles and let it fly. It was hard to believe this was the same little boy whom I implored to "water a tree" last summer in a similar emergency situation, and he absolutely refused. (I ended up pounding on the door of a local restaurant in Senoia—about two hours before they were open for business—and they generously allowed Krischan to use the restroom. His comment as we left: "This restaurant must not be any good because there aren't any customers.")

All I can figure is it must have been the pressure of running his first race. I asked him as we headed to the starting line what made him so bold; he didn't have an explanation, but as we got close to the gathering of runners he asked me if we could stop talking about this now? After all, it was time to get down to business. Besides, it wasn't a good idea for G-Pa's to embarrass their grandsons when they were about to compete in an athletic competition for the first time.

As we waited at the back of a pack of 100 or so runners (the 5K and the one-mile started simultaneously, but the two races took different routes), I told Krischan not to start out too fast because, after all, a mile is a really long way. Over the years Krischan has covered as many as three miles with me, but as you might imagine not all of it was running. There was always a good amount of walking, talking to neighbors, and petting every dog that crossed our path. But today would be different: Today was all about *running.*

As the race director was going over the instructions for the races, Krischan asked if we could hold hands while we ran. "You know, so you can keep up with me, G-Pa." I told him he would need to have his hands free so he could pump his arms as he ran, but I would do my absolute best to keep up with him.

Krischan started off exactly as I asked: conservative pace, arms-a-pumping, and cheeks turning bright red as he crested the first of several hills on one of the more challenging fun-run courses I've ever seen. Let me be the first to say the experience was wonderful: He smiled the entire time, slowed down only for a couple of steps because his stomach hurt, and even managed to squeeze in a little exploration and housekeeping along the way. Krischan waved to everyone along the course and got excited every time someone shouted him encouragement. ("Do they know me, G-Pa? They must because they're cheering for me!")

We played leapfrog with several other runners for most of the race. As you probably already guessed I took my fair share of photos along the way so I could have a record of this special morning. As we neared the finish line, by my calculation we were in the middle of a pack of about 25 runners, walkers, moms, dads, and one lone G-Pa. I told Krischan he should cross the finish line in front of me because I wasn't wearing a number, but he would have none of it. We would be crossing the finish line together. I think what he said was "Catch up to me, G-Pa; I'll slow down so you can," which was his subtle way of reminding me I'm not as young as him (he thinks I'm 25, by the way).

We ran the final 10 or so glorious steps together and crossed Krischan's first finish line in an official time of eighteen minutes and twelve seconds. 18:12, a time that is now part of my vernacular along with 76:36 (a 10-mile race Josh ran when he was nine years old), 3:18:15 (Cindy's first half-marathon), and 36:14 (my 10K best). I imagine when my memory starts failing me—I'm guessing around the time I'm running my great-grandchild's first race with him or her—the time I'll still remember will be 18:12.

While Krischan may not remember his finishing time, I have high hopes that he'll always remember the day he ran just like his G-Pa.

Postscript: Six weeks later I paced Krischan in his second one-mile race. He ran—all 5,280 feet—and lowered his time by almost six minutes, finishing in 12 minutes and 21 seconds. The next time out he lowered his time to 11 minutes and 11 seconds.

It won't be long before he'll be running faster than his G-Pa.

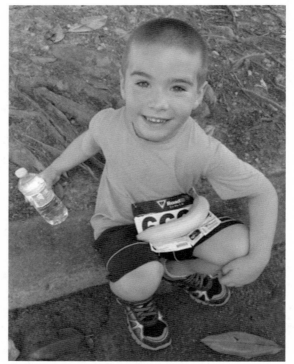

Krischan after his first official race in Griffin, Georgia

IN MY SKIN

OCTOBER 2014

It's no secret I run every single day, which qualifies me as a "streaker." What remains a secret to most everyone except for a very small circle of friends is that I am also a streaker. Yes, that means exactly what you think it means: I have run nekkid.

Although almost 40 years have passed since those ten minutes of alcohol-induced spontaneity that took me on a circuitous route from my dormitory room through the women's dormitory next door and around the Arts and Sciences building (where ironically four years later I would have an office on the second floor as a Graduate Teaching Assistant) and then through the Rathskellar (the on-campus bar) and finally up three flights of stairs back to where I started. I must mention I had an accomplice: My dorm-mate and best friend from high school was with me—every sip and every step of the way. I was 18 years old and as you probably already surmised common sense was the furthest thing from my mind.

Four decades later I'm not the same person I was in college. I've gained a lot of wisdom and common sense over the years (although my wife might suggest otherwise) and now run every day wearing clothes.

Except today, that is.

Early this morning, as I did as a freshman at the University of Florida on a rather chilly Friday night in the fall so long ago, I ran along the streets of _____ (city/state/country intentionally omitted to prevent possible criminal action in the future) wearing nothing but a pair of New Balance running shoes and a smile (and a flashlight to alert oncoming cars that I was running along the side of the road). Originally, I wanted to run naked legally; I was planning to run in a race at a nudist colony in north Georgia last spring. In the past I had been invited by the race director—more than once, as a matter of fact—to run in the Fig Leaf 5K but decided against it each time, seeing as I had all of this wisdom and common sense swelling up inside of me and all. But this year I decided it was time to give it a try, but by the time I inquired about it the race had already been held. I missed it by a couple of days, which led me to where I was this morning: Running along the streets of _____ (irritating, isn't it?) on a dark _____ (chilly, warm, tepid, foggy, rainy, windy—conditions intentionally omitted; you know why) morning...butt nekkid.

OK, so I didn't run the entire 10 miles this morning that way. I ran a few miles, removed everything I was wearing but my shoes, and ran a good 10 minutes or so down the road with only three concerns in mind: whether or not I would be recognized, arrested, or experience any pain caused by (for lack of a better term) "package slappage."

Ten minutes into the "natural" portion of my run I was ready to turn around and head back: Back to my pile of stashed clothing, back to where I started running *au natural*, and back to reality. But then the thought occurred to me: to be truly at one with nature my feet should be touching Mother Earth. Besides, I was thinking back to earlier this year when I spent the day with my grandson, and he wanted me to take him running. I noticed he was wearing flip-flops and told him he couldn't run in them. He insisted on running, so I asked him what he would be running in since all he had was flip-flops. I can still hear his reply: In my feet.

So with one shoe in either hand I ran the last 10 minutes of my *au natural* run, stopping only to pull the occasional impediment (pebble/piece of glass/Kryptonite—hard to tell in the dark) out of my foot. It made me think back to when I lived in Hawaii and wearing shoes was the exception rather than the rule. Over the course of the three years I lived on Oahu the bottoms of my feet developed a leathery almost reptilian quality to them—a time when I didn't give a second thought to walking barefoot on broken glass. But my feet couldn't compare to the feet of the legendary Randall Tanaka, a classmate of mine at Moanalua Intermediate School. Randall's feet were so tough he could walk barefoot through fire, a fact I know to be true because I saw him do it. I was the Senior Patrol Leader of our Boy Scout Troop, and after a Tuesday night meeting we built a campfire to roast marshmallows and a few other objects I don't care to talk about here. Randall boasted to some of the Scouts he could stand barefoot on the open fire for as long as it took to toast a marshmallow, and after just the right amount of laughter—and wagering—he hopped into the fire and stepped from one burning log to the next while everyone else literally sat around the campfire with their mouths wide open and the blankest of stares on their faces as Randall told them to "pay up, suckers!" On the way home from the meeting Randall and I stopped at a department store and he used his winnings to buy a box of 24 giant Sweet Tarts, one of the four major food groups of Troop #201.

Interesting aside: In my entire career in both Cub and Boy Scouts I went camping only once. It was my first year in Cub Scouts in Quonset Point, Rhode Island. It was only one night alone in the woods, but it left considerable emotional scars. I built a lean-to

*in which to sleep and store my belongings. If you're not familiar
with a lean-to I suggest you watch the first episode of any given
season of* Survivor *and see what the tribes build out of branches
and palm fronds for shelter. What you'll see makes the castaways
of* Gilligan's Island *look like the Frank Lloyd Wrights of island ar-
chitecture. The only difference between the huts built by the con-
testants on* Survivor *and my lean-to is this: Their huts have roofs
that leak while my lean-to was open on one side and allowed four
inches of snow to accumulate during the night. It makes me wonder how I ever made Senior Patrol Leader, a fact I find almost as
ironic as putting the finishing touches on a graduate degree within the walls of a building I had run around bare-a** naked a few
years earlier.*

So once I got back to my pile of clothes on the side of the road and
dressed in total darkness (try to distinguish between your right
shoe and your left shoe in the dark sometime; not as easy as you
might think), I headed back to _____ (come on; you didn't
think I was going to slip up NOW, did you?) and hopped in the
shower, wondering whether or not I would ever mention what I'd
done over the past 90 minutes.

And now you're well aware what I decided to do: Write it down
for the world to see!

Maybe my wife has the right idea after all. I may be a little light
on the wisdom and common sense, but I'm also pretty light on my
feet.

Especially when I'm not wearing any clothes.

AGING GRACEFULLY

NOVEMBER 2014

It started over 20 years ago. On my 40th birthday I ran 40 miles. On my 45th birthday I ran 45 miles. This went on for another decade (in five year/mile increments) until I decided that 55 miles on my 55th birthday was a good place to call a truce between my aging body and this 20-year tradition. That, or at the very least convert to kilometers on my 60th birthday (that would mean running 37.2 miles for anyone not fluent in metric).

As I've come to learn, time has a way of sneaking up on you. I'll be 60 this December and it was time to make a decision. It took all of 60 seconds:

I wanted to run 60 miles; kilometers are for wimps (sorry, Europe).

The first thing I needed was an accomplice. *What's that, Sarah? You just ran your first 100-miler this summer, you're hungry for more, and all I have to do is say when? Give me a couple of dates that work for you, and I'll see which days I have available, and we'll go from there.*

Once Sarah and I agreed that Sunday, November 16, would work for both of us I got an email with the volunteer schedule for church. My wife Cindy and I were scheduled to work at Grand Central (the information counter) on November 16. I asked Kathi the scheduler to swap me out with someone on November 23 and asked that she not tell Cindy about my plans to run 60 miles on the 16th.

So what happens next? Cindy comes home one evening and says she saw a revised Grand Central schedule and that I was no longer scheduled to work with her on the 16th. I said I asked Kathi to schedule me for the 23rd as I had something to do on the 16th.

Cindy: Kathi said you were running a race. Are you going out of town?

Me: No. I'll be here.

Cindy: Are you going to be running?

Me: Yes.

Cindy: And it's going to take most of the day?

Me: Yes.

Cindy: Well, it's not your birthday.

Me: But it's *almost* my birthday.

Cindy: Oh Lord, please don't tell me you're running 60 miles.

Me: OK, I won't.

(Insert sound of a lead balloon hitting the ground)

Cindy knows me all too well. I think in her heart she knew 60 miles was inevitable, although she was probably hoping and praying I would at the very least convert to the metric system once I reached decade number 6.

As the date drew nearer the usual suspects lined up to run some of the miles with me. Al, Susan, Val, Eric, Sarah, and my son Josh said they'd join me to give me the best birthday gift they could possibly offer: themselves.

I laid out a flat (well, at least it seemed flat when I drove it in my truck), shaded 2.5-mile route starting and finishing in downtown Haralson (population zero, although it is a very familiar locale to anyone who watches the opening credits to *The Walking Dead*). The plan was to run the loop 24 times counterclockwise beginning at 6 a.m. My friends could join me any time throughout the day. Their instructions: Look for my blue Gator truck in deserted, downtown Haralson and wait—I'll be coming by about every 27 minutes for the first 35 miles or so, but after that all bets were off. I hoped to finish up around 6 p.m. if everything went according to plan.

Sarah and Josh started with me at (officially) 6:02 a.m. Josh, getting a little exposure to an ultrarunning endeavor, studied the assorted food and drink I loaded on the back of the truck: Gatorade, water, soda, chocolate milk, ginger snaps, and pretzels—all things I would soon be sick of and wouldn't eat or drink for weeks after today. We used a flashlight for the first loop as we took note of the solitude and the incredibly great weather we were blessed with (40 degrees, slight breeze, overcast). Josh ran 10 miles and then headed home as he was going to church with Cindy. I made note that Josh stopped to answer Nature's Call about every three miles, lending more support to the apple not falling far from the tree theory. Sarah held on for 25 miles before calling it a day, but by that time Eric had shown up wanting to run 20 miles so it looked like I'd have company for at least the first 45 miles of my run.

Now would be a good time to interject what didn't happen during the course of the day:

- I didn't trip and fall.

- I didn't have to stop to answer Nature's *Other* Call.

- I didn't change clothes (although I did remove my jacket after the first loop).

- I didn't change shoes.

- I didn't cuss (although Eric said I exhaled the word "sh*t" every other breath).

- I didn't have any close encounters with mean dogs or hostile Haralsonians.

- I didn't quit. (Wanted to, but didn't. More on that shortly.)

Al and Susan showed up for their 10 miles shortly after Eric started running with me. Once Eric completed his 20 miles and called it a day, I still had six more ibuprofen remaining before my run was complete. (Let me explain: I counted off 24 ibuprofen—one for each of the laps I needed to run—and placed them on the right side of the back bumper on the truck. After each lap I would move one ibuprofen to the left side of the bumper; once all 24 had made it from one side to the other I would be finished. My only concern was that someone might show up while I was in the middle of a loop, consume a couple of the ibuprofen and forget which pile they took them from.)

I ran briskly for the next three laps once Eric left (no one was with me to tell you anything different, so yes I RAN BRISKLY FOR THE NEXT THREE LAPS). Toward the end of my 21st lap I heard a car approaching me from behind: It was Val. She was finished showing houses for the day and could go home (she lives about three miles away) and change into her running attire if I wanted company for the final three laps. If she only knew what was running through my head during that 21st lap (52.5 miles isn't bad, is it? Who could fault me if I stopped? Etc., etc.), she wouldn't have needed to ask.

Fifteen minutes later she returned, and the two of us ran, walked, reminisced (Val and I have been friends so long that she was by my side when I ran my 40th mile on my 40th birthday, and I was by her side three weeks later when she ran her 35th mile on her 35th birthday), and laughed—yes, *LAUGHED*—until the last three ibuprofen made it to the left side of the bumper.

I looked at my watch when we finished: 6:12 p.m. We shared a couple of beers I had hidden in the cooler beneath the two 64-ounce bottles of Gatorade and 20 pounds of ice. Pitch black evening (you couldn't see the stars for the cloud cover), total silence, deserted town of Haralson—boarded up buildings everywhere—and two old friends sharing a beer after doing what they loved doing most. Val hit the nail on the head when she referred to it as 'surreal,' because it most certainly was.

I took the following day as a vacation day from work. After all, I'm not a 52-year-old kid anymore (and the mere fact that I refer to someone 52 or 53 as a kid sort of tells you something about me), and I knew I'd need the day to recover.

That next morning—after my two cups of coffee, of course—I took a personal inventory of which parts of my body hurt. Here's a short list:

- Everything.

Al has been encouraging me for years—starting about the time I was still a 52-year-old kid—that I should learn to cut back my mileage, stop running so hard, and age gracefully. Now that I've gotten this 60-miler out of my system I'm ready to do just that.

Note to Val: Thanks for pulling me through those last three loops. I don't think I could have done them without you. I'm sorry I won't be in town in a few weeks for your birthday. That is, unless you're ready to convert to kilometers. Then we'll talk.

Postscript: Two weeks later—on Sunday, November 30, 2014—I ran. The day was the 36-year anniversary of the day I started a streak of running every day. Two weeks after that I ran the Tallahassee Ultra Distance Classic 50K...and ran 10 additional kilometers to bookend my birthday run: 60 miles on the front and 60 kilometers on the back. What the heck: I did the same thing when I turned 40 and 50. I promise not to do it again at 70.

Post-Postscript: Four weeks later I ran the Jacksonville Marathon, thereby giving me a marathon finish in five decades (20s, 30s, 40s, 50s, and now 60s). My friend Al turns 70 next May. He also has run a marathon in five decades. The ball is now in his court.

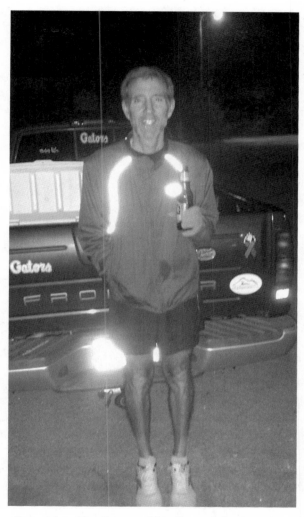

Scott after 60 miles...and his first celebratory beer

THE TIME IS NOW

NOVEMBER 2014

November 29, 1978.

People were anxious to see what JR would do next on *Dallas*.

Lord of the Rings—the **original** *Lord of the Rings*—was ruling the box office.

Donna Summer's *MacArthur Park* was in heavy rotation on the radio, and all the popular discotheques. (Yes, you heard me: Discotheques!)

A new car sold for $6,400, and its 16-gallon gas tank could be filled for a little over $10.

I had been married a little over a year, attending graduate school at the University of Florida, living in married student housing, and teaching two public speaking courses to undergraduates. Lou Ann Fernald was in my first period class (more on that later).

November 29, 1978. It was also the last day I didn't run.

I started running every day on Thursday, November 30, 1978— less than two weeks before I took my oral exams for my master's degree with the two professors who had gotten me interested in running several months earlier. I didn't run the previous day because I spent the day in the bathroom, the result of winning a bet with one of my professors. What was the bet, you ask?

Me: *I can run 13 miles.*

Professor: *I bet you can't.*

I won the bet. That is, if you consider running 13 miles for the first time and then spending the next day never more than 20 feet away from the toilet because your stomach felt as if it had been mauled by a grizzly bear as winning, then yes, I won the bet.

Today is Sunday, November 30, 2014. I'll be turning 60 in 10 days. I've been pounding the pavement to the tune of 137,000 miles over the past 36 years. There was a 16-year period in my life when I averaged a half marathon a day. OK, I admit a minor addiction to running lots and lots of miles and have resolved each of the last 20 years to cut back (without fail, I might add), but today I'm going to do something about it.

After all, 36 years of averaging more than 10 miles a day and knocking on the door of my 60th birthday is as good a time as any to start thinking about some of the things I want to be able to do in the years ahead, such as:

- Negotiate the stairs down to the basement and up to the bonus room on the second level of our new home.

- Chase my grandson through the woods, up and down the driveway, and all around the back yard.

- Carry a 42-pound bag of kitty litter from the trunk of the car to the basement.

- Rake almost two acres' worth of leaves in the fall.

- Roll a full garbage can down our 300-foot long driveway every Tuesday morning, and then pull the empty garbage can back *up* the driveway on Tuesday afternoon.

You get the idea.

Long story short: My body is tired. Once the sun goes down—whether its daylight saving time or not—I'm ready to call it a day and turn in for the night. Sad but true.

So today is the beginning of the New Me. I'm not going to feel compelled to run 9 or 10 miles every weekday. I won't feel obligated to run considerably longer distances on weekends. I'm not...I won't...I'm ready to ***JUST SAY NO*** to high mileage.

Now if you'll excuse me, I have to ask the Old Me to explain to the New Me why we ran 13 miles this morning. Once we're both on the same page I know we'll be just fine. Starting tomorrow.

Getting back to Lou Ann Fernald, six months after taking my class she went on to bigger and better things as *Playboy* magazine's Miss June 1979.

As for me, it's now 36 years later, and my body has never graced the pages of *Runner's World.*

But there's always tomorrow.

LAST CALL AT WAKULLA

DECEMBER 2014

From my experience, I've known runners to be creatures of habit. They find a brand of running shoes that provide the comfort and support they need and use them exclusively if not religiously. They blaze a favorite trail known only to them and run it again and again until they're able to know what time it is simply by realizing where they are on the route at any given time. They discover a drink or a snack—sometimes both that has served them well during their runs and refuse to try anything else.

And if that runner is anything like me, they find a race they really enjoy and die a thousand deaths when that race is no more.

The first race falling into that category was the Olander Park 24-Hour Run, held on a shaded 1.09-mile asphalt path around a beautiful lake in Sylvania, Ohio. Race director Tom Falvey had the unique ability of making everyone feel like a champion. The runner who completed 50 miles in 24 hours was given the same accolades as the winner who ran more than 150. Over time the number of entrants no longer supported the expenses for conducting the 24-Hour Run, so in 2003 it was turned into a 100-mile event. I ran it twice more and then—in the blink of an eye—it was gone. However, the memories remain. In its 24-hour format, completing 129 miles in 2002 which helped me land an invitation to the 2003 Badwater Ultramarathon. As a 100-mile event, running with my friend Gary Griffin in 2004 and seeing him finish his first 100-miler, and then Gary and me running it again in 2005 when we both saw mutual friend Susan Lance finish *her* first 100-miler.

The second race that fell by the wayside was the Atlanta Marathon. Since 1981 I had spent every Thanksgiving morning lining up for the South's oldest marathon until it was taken away—cold turkey, no less—in 2010. Out of respect I ran the marathon course on Thanksgiving morning for several more years after that until I grew weary of running on a route filled with unchaperoned holiday morning traffic in busy downtown Atlanta.

Last year I said my goodbyes to the good people at Brooks Elementary School in Brooks, Georgia, as their PTO put on the 31st and final edition of the Brooks Day 10K. I'll miss so much about this quaint little race held in conjunction with the Brooks Day Festival on the second Saturday in May: walking the halls of the school to use the restroom one last time before the race and seeing all the students' drawings and paintings proudly displayed on the bulletin boards, attending the awards presentation and listening for the names of the runners I ran with every weekend as they were called to the main stage to receive their awards, and heading over to the festivities in the park afterward to watch the young kids play T-ball while enjoying a hot, fresh funnel cake courtesy of one of the local merchants.

This December I'll be heading down to the Florida panhandle to run in the Tallahassee Ultra Distance Classic (TUDC). Next year the race moves to a new venue, and I want to enjoy the cozy confines of Wakulla Springs State Park—where it's been held since I fell in love with it the very first time I ran it back in 1998—one last time. The quiet seclusion and natural beauty the park offers will take a back seat on the second Saturday in December however, because that's when the ultrarunning community gathers in Wakulla for its annual family reunion and "run through the jungle" (as the event has been called in recent years) for the last time.

In my 17-year love affair with the TUDC the event had been directed by two husband-and-wife teams whose organization and attention to detail was surpassed only by their commitment to the sport of running and shared passion for making sure each and every runner had the best ultra experience possible. (On how many race applications have you been asked to name your favorite aid station refreshments?) I was welcomed to Wakulla by then-race directors Fred and Margarete Deckert that first time and when the event was passed along to current race directors Gary and Peg Griffin (that would be the same Gary Griffin who ran his first 100-miler with me back in 2004). I'm happy to report nothing was lost in translation. (Next year when the torch is passed along to Jeff and JoLena Bryan I trust that will be the case as well.) The TUDC remains a first-class event, but more importantly it continues to be a family affair.

The host Gulf Winds Track Club always has plenty of members on hand to provide support. Enthusiastically calling out your name as you finish a lap* and meticulously notating your split time on a clipboard, carefully filling your bottle full of your favorite sports drink, or enthusiastically running a lap with you because you need an emotional lift, they do it all. Hot soup, free massages and awards created by local artists are available after you've finished with your 50-kilometers or 50-miles (your choice!). From my personal experience—10 trips to Wakulla and almost 400 miles of running there—I can honestly say I've never made a request that wasn't granted (including the year I asked a volunteer to take down my Darkside Running Club banner because I'd just spent more than eight hours running 50-miles in monsoon conditions and 41-degree temperatures).

---

* *Originally one lap was an intimate 2.07-mile route through the park. In 2010, it was modified to a 10-kilometer route, much of it outside of the confines of Wakulla Springs State Park.*

The Tallahassee Ultra Distance Classic has a storied history (do yourself a favor and research it on the internet when you have some time) and is the proud home of numerous record-setting performances and countless first-time ultra-finishers. On a personal level, I've forged many personal relationships at Wakulla that have stood the test of time as well as the endless miles we've run together over the years.

I have many fond memories of my 10 trips to Wakulla Springs State Park. When I return to the Wakulla Lodge this year to run the TUDC one last time I have no doubt that each and every one of them will run through my mind at some point during the weekend. (I always make the TUDC a weekend adventure, driving down on Friday and driving home on Sunday.)

The memory that stands out most is that second Saturday in December in 2007. I had just lost both of my parents within a period of six weeks prior to the TUDC and thought—although I wasn't particularly keen on running 31 miles—that being around some familiar faces would do me good. Fifteen minutes prior to the start, race director Gary gave his usual spirited and motivational pre-race speech and ended it by dedicating the race to the memories of my mom and dad. Then once the race began I ran the first couple of laps with Amy Costa, who offered me an eight-mile-per-hour shoulder to lean on as she spoke about how much her father meant to her before transitioning to asking me questions about my parents. I couldn't have paid for better therapy.

Come to find out I was exactly right: Being around some familiar faces did me good.

Especially when the familiar faces were those of my family.

Postscript: After the race co-race director Gary Griffin sent the following message:

At the onset of the race last Saturday it seemed that this would be the final Tallahassee Ultra Distance Classic to ever take place at the hallowed venue of Wakulla Springs State Park. But while you were out there running, something quite unexpected and wonderfully exciting happened...your basic Christmas miracle, if you will. Nancy Stedman and Jay Silvania, the outgoing and longtime RDs of the Tallahassee Marathon, offered to assume directorship of the 2015 TUDC at Wakulla Springs. Jeff and JoLena Bryan, who were the Gulf Winds Track Club Board-approved RDs for the 2015 TUDC will now become the RDs of a local 8-hour run in 2015 at a place and date to be determined. This is all subject to board approval, but at this point it certainly appears as though the long history of the TUDC at Wakulla Springs on the 2nd Saturday in December will continue!

Footnote: When I posted my "Last Call at Wakulla" story on my Facebook page the first one to "like" it was Jay Silvania. My work is done.

BURNING BRIDGES

DECEMBER 2014

Buckman. Fuller Warren. Acosta. Dames Point. Mathews. These are the names of a few of the many bridges you'll find in Jacksonville, Florida.

If you want to visit Jacksonville you're inevitably going to cross the St. Johns River at some point.

Main Street. Hart. If you're going to run in Jacksonville's top running event, the Gate River Run, you'll be crossing the river via these two bridges. On foot, of course.

I've run the race 10 times. I ran my first 15K at the River Run. I ran my fastest 15K there, arguably the best race I've ever run. At one time, it was my favorite race.

I've also been to Jacksonville to run the marathon no less than nine times. At one time the race finished in downtown Jacksonville; the route included the crossing of two bridges, one early in the race and one late in the race. I ran my first Boston qualifier in Jacksonville. I've run my personal best there as well.

The current route of the Jacksonville Marathon doesn't include any bridges. The course is as flat as week-old roadkill. I ran this year's race and was surprised to find myself red-faced, embarrassed, and totally exhausted. What's even more surprising is that all of this happened 15 hours prior to the start of the race: At the packet pick-up where I picked up my race bib (number).

Let me explain.

I signed up for the marathon back in June. Early registration was $70, a relative bargain in today's world of ever-increasing entry fees. (In comparison this year's New York City Marathon cost $255 to enter; $347 for non-U.S. residents.) I sent my application and a personal check through the U.S. mail. My friend Valerie—who entered the race on a whim at the last minute—well after I signed up—and I went to the 1st Place Sports Running store on Baymeadows Road to pick up our race packets. Incidentally, I've brought many a runner to the Jacksonville races over the years; the significance of that comment will be apparent shortly.

We checked the printed list of entrants in the store's parking lot to find our corresponding race numbers so we could ask for our respective packets. Val spotted her name immediately and had her number in hand while I was still scouring the list for mine. It became evident after five or six minutes that my name simply was not on the list.

I was directed to the go inside the store where I was handed off to Jane Alred, who just so happens to be the wife of the marathon's race director. (I assure you I had no intention of using her name; however, as you will soon understand why I told her I intended to write about this experience in the very near future, and she handed me her business card so I could subsequently spell her name correctly.)

Jane asked me if I had proof that I registered for the marathon. Well, let's see: I had the original application in hand that clearly shows I detached the mail-in application, I drove all the way down from Atlanta to participate, and I've been running races in

Jacksonville for well over 30 years. Most of all—plain and simple—I'm telling you that I did.

Sorry, not good enough. Jane asked me if I had the canceled check for the entry fee. I explained that my bank didn't send canceled checks with the monthly statement, and I really didn't know. "Well, here's what you can do: You can pay the early entry fee again and once you prove you already registered I'll refund your money."

Now it was my turn: "Sorry, not good enough." Val told me later she could tell how upset I was because my face was beet red (actually what she said was "as red as my chicken's wattles and comb when they get mad" but I have no idea what that means). Val added that anyone could tell I was being completely honest by the conviction in my voice and face. Apparently anyone except Jane, that is.

Jane went to the back room and returned with a cardboard box containing the applications that had been mailed in. There couldn't have been more than 50 in an event that encompassed thousands. Mine wasn't in there. "The U.S. mail isn't always perfect; maybe they returned your entry." I assured her they didn't. She assured me she didn't receive my entry and didn't "want my money twice," although earlier she asked for my money twice because I knew with absolute certainty I mailed my application, and she already had my money once.

I told her I was a race director myself, and if the roles were reversed I would believe her without hesitation and grant her request in a heartbeat. I told her I've always known runners to be the most honorable people in the world.

She replied that she'd been taken advantage of—many times, in fact—over the years, and it wasn't going to happen again.

Being the hothead, I can be when I know I am absolutely right, I said "fine, I'll just run without a number." Jane shrugged and walked off. (I want to mention I did not have my checkbook with me, and I wasn't about to give her my credit card information that she promised to refund once she received proof of my "alleged" earlier payment. Seriously, if they lost/misplaced/whatever my application, what were the chances I would get my credit card refund?)

That's when cooler heads prevailed. Val asked me to call my wife Cindy and ask her to go online and check our bank statements. I knew Cindy had a really busy weekend and wasn't sure she would even have the password with her (she was working at her store at the time), but I called anyway. Miracle of miracles: Cindy found the canceled check online (cashed on June 17), scanned a photo of it, and sent it to my cell phone. I, in turn, sent it to Val's tablet which I took to Jane who in turn asked me to follow her outside where she hand wrote my information and gave me a number for the marathon…without the slightest hint of an apology. I repeat: Without the slightest hint of an apology, although she continued to try to convince me she didn't want to take my money twice and how some people can be so dishonest.

Backstory: Several years ago, a friend of mine was running competitively for the Atlanta Track Club at the Gate River Run. She called me the day before the race and explained that she was given a back-of-the-pack number rather than a seeded number (reserved for faster runners so they can start at the front of the race) and needed my help. I wrote the race director (Jane's husband, remember?) and vouched for my friend's credentials as an established and talented runner. He took me at my word and gave my friend a seeded number while I took comfort that my reputation in the world of running meant something. Heck, a similar testimonial from the office of the Atlanta Track Club on my friend's behalf moments earlier had fallen on deaf ears, thus the request to me.

After giving everything I possibly have to give to the sport of running for these past 36-plus years I didn't deserve to be treated the way I was at 1st Place Sports. Factoring in the absence of an apology only made matters worse. Again, if the roles were reversed I would have offered her the sincerest of apologies once I was proven wrong. Not only wrong, but dead wrong.

It got me to thinking about a lot of things. I woke up the next morning at 1:30 a.m. and spent the next four hours thinking about these very words you are reading right now. What could possibly have made Jane treat me the way she did? What triggered her comment about being taken advantage of?

Then I thought of something I've said (as well as written) many, many times: *Runners are some of the finest people I've ever known.* Could I have been wrong all this time?

Then this thought dawned on me: Road races—particularly marathons and ultras—are charging more and more money every year for the simple privilege of running in them. I have a difficult time believing these costs are justifiable, yet here we are. Why do the big-name and big-ticket events charge outrageous entry fees for their events? I can't help but think the answer is—plain and simple—because people will pay them.

Most people, that is. It's entirely possible that some runners have had to resort to fabricating stories about "lost applications" to finagle their way into a race they desperately want to run—that special race charging an exorbitant entry fee, money that could be put to better use toward other things. Food, clothing, and shelter for example; things a little more important than a three-dollar finisher's medal or a race shirt listing all its sponsors on the back.

So perhaps the way Jane treated me wasn't the reason I found myself red-faced, embarrassed, and totally exhausted before the Jacksonville Marathon even began. Maybe the real reason is something that has been bothering me for the last 10 years: race directors that are more interested in making a buck than taking care of their runners.

That's why I've always been fond of the races in Jacksonville: sensible entry fees and a passionate concern for the welfare of the runners.

That's why it saddens me to say I won't be returning to Jacksonville to run either the Jacksonville Marathon or the Gate River Run ever again.

Those bridges across the St. Johns are now engulfed in flames.

2015

GOING OUT WITH BOTH BARRELS BLAZING

THE NEXT CHAPTER

JANUARY 2015

You all know her as Anne Rentz. I've called her "Chapter One" for the last six years, a reference to Anne being the subject of the first chapter in my book, *A Passion for Running*. The title of Anne's chapter is "Running for Fun" and depicts the transformation of an admitted couch potato at 40 years of age taking up the sport of running and then taking her life in an entirely new direction—one of exercise, physical fitness, and eventually the finish line of a 100-mile race.

Anne's transformation from couch potato to athlete began when she lived in Marietta, Georgia, and ventured outside one day for a casual walk. She met up with a group of people who told her they walked every day; they invited Anne to join them. One member of the group was a William Mayfield Cox, Jr., who had lived his entire life in Marietta. It wasn't long before "Eagle Bill" became a large part of Anne's life. Friend, coach, mentor...and then 15 years later, husband.

Anne and Bill were married for a little over seven years before Bill's life on earth sadly and suddenly came to an end. The date: January 12, 2015. He was 83 years young and only a few months removed from fulfilling his dream of riding the 95 miles of the Silver Comet Trail on his recumbent tricycle. Bill's late-in-life accomplishment is not surprising. At age 55 he suffered a heart attack and his doctor advised him to exercise if he wanted to continue living. Bill took the doctor's advice to heart. He immediately started walking four miles every day, and his commitment to a healthy lifestyle served him well for the next three decades.

Bill lived quite the full life. As Anne's sister Becky said so eloquently at his memorial service, Bill was "the wind beneath Anne's wings." He was also:

- President of Cox Printing Company in Marietta for 60 years

- Little League coach of the Westside Warriors football team

- President and coach of Custer Park baseball

- Founding member of the Circle of Wisdom Social Club

- Member of the First United Church

- Committed husband, father, grandfather, and brother

Bill's belief in physical fitness and an active lifestyle was exemplified not only by his involvement as a competitor, coach, and enthusiast but also through his volunteerism. It was a regular sight for many years to see Bill supporting Anne in her races of marathon distances or longer while doing all he could to support the other competitors as well. In 2008 Bill earned the Darkside Running Club's Mama Betty Award, a recognition bestowed on the outstanding volunteer of the year.

It is my honor to have known Bill Cox as a friend. I don't ever recall seeing him without his infectious smile, a hat on his head, or Anne by his side. As those who know him can attest, Bill was never at a loss for words. The man loved to talk. He also loved his family, he loved his country, and he loved his Chapter One.

My favorite photo of Bill and Anne is on page 272 of *A Passion for Running*. Both of them have smiles on their faces (shockingly, Bill isn't wearing a hat) and cutting a piece of their wedding cake hand-in-hand. The caption beneath the picture reads, "Bill and Anne, Husband and Wife."

I encourage you to look at that photo so you can see the smile on Bill's face.

Then you can appreciate something I've always known: Anne was the wind beneath Bill's wings as well.

You will be missed, Eagle Bill. Missed, but never forgotten.

RUNNING FREE

JANUARY 2015

My first official pair of running shoes cost $5. They weren't one of the top brands at the time—Nike or Onitsuka Tiger were the ones costing the big bucks—but they were honest-to-goodness running shoes. I bought them at Marty Liquori's original Athletic Attic store in Gainesville, Florida. When I wore them for the first time I couldn't possibly have been more excited, especially after running my first 30 or 40 miles in a pair of Stan Smith tennis shoes.

My first official race entry fee—Leonardo's Lap, a five-mile event sponsored by a local pizza parlor in Gainesville—cost $3. There was pizza and beer at the finish line and a really cool race T-shirt that I proudly wore for many, many years. The fact that I still remember my finishing time (36:32 if you're interested) should indicate how special crossing that first finishing line meant to me.

The first time I drank Gatorade I paid nine cents. It came in a 32-ounce glass bottle and was available in two flavors: lemon-lime and orange. Drinking Gatorade made me feel like an athlete. Not just an athlete, but a *runner.*

The year was 1978. Running was fun. Running was simple. And without a doubt, running was inexpensive. The most expensive running item at the time was a lifetime subscription to *Runner's World* that could be purchased for $200 which was a small fortune at that time, especially for a newlywed graduate teaching assistant.

Times have changed and boy-oh-boy how the cost of running has changed.

Let me start with a $169 pair of running shoes that the manufacturer would have you believe makes you "fly." If you believe what a manufacturer will tell you—that running shoes should be retired every 500 miles or so—every three miles you run in those $169 shoes will cost you $1, thus making a car or truck a more economical mode of transportation than running. (By the way, it's not unusual for me to put 2,000 miles on a single pair of shoes. I've never been one to listen to the so-called experts, which may explain why *Runner's World* never kept my interest.)

Then there's the high-profile marathons held in the major cities that will set you back several hundred dollars just for a spot on the starting line. Beyond that the likelihood you'll need an airline ticket (have you priced airline tickets lately?), lodging (some of you may have noticed how local hotels raise their rates when runners come to town), and any other incidentals (dining, memorabilia at the marathon expo, post-race celebratory drinks) you'll be inclined to spend your hard-earned dollars on. If experience has taught me anything, it's that runners in general have a real propensity to be loose with the purse strings when they're caught up in the atmosphere of a major race.

I've seen running shorts that cost as much as a pair of Nike or Onitsuka Tigers used to cost. Actually, it's more like three times as much, sometimes as much as four.

Don't get me wrong. If you're comfortable spending that much money on running shoes, running attire, and race entry fees— and if you can afford it—then more power to you. I can't tell you that I didn't spend a pretty penny on the like myself over the years, but I will tell you the time has come for the madness to stop. My running and my wallet need to come to an understanding.

I buy last year's running shoes when the shelves are cleared off to make room for this year's models so last years' are sold at rock-bottom prices. I'm very selective in the races I run and as a general rule of thumb I stick to the low-key races that offer affordable entry fees, volunteers that make you feel appreciated, and the personal satisfaction of feeling like I'm more than just a (bib) number. I wear running shorts until the elastic around the waist band begins stretching out instead of pulling in.

I don't need shoes that make me feel like I can fly. I refuse to spend money on an entry fee that could otherwise be spent on groceries that could feed my family for several weeks (yes—weeks). I don't care if the shorts I'm wearing were worn for the first time a decade ago.

Don't fall prey to following the masses. Do what YOU want to do. There is no one you need to impress other than yourself. Don't buy the latest, greatest pair of running shoes because everyone else is buying them. New shoes won't make you run any faster than your old shoes, let alone fly. Don't feel obligated to spend a small fortune to run an event simply because that's what all the cool kids are doing. Be your own person, because after all that's a large part of what makes you a runner.

Running isn't about wearing the most expensive shoes, the latest attire, or the trendiest gadget (does anyone really believe a device can tell you how many calories you've burned?). Running isn't about spending several thousand dollars to run *the* race...and *the* race after that and *the* race after that. Running isn't all about spending money.

Rather, running is all about freedom. All you need is a comfortable pair of running shoes, modest attire suitable for the conditions, and a wide-open country road or secluded trail where you can run free. The best thing about freedom is—*surprise!*—it's free. Is this a great country or what?

Free of the desk where you spend more than 40 hours a week. Free from the stress that consumes the majority of your every waking hour. Free from traffic, telemarketers, and television. Free from everything you want—and *need*—to be free of.

I'll admit I've spent my fair share of money on my running habit over the years. I'm now at the point in life where the most rewarding runs are those that begin in my driveway and end at my mailbox. When I have the opportunity to spend some time in my favorite places I always make time to run some of my favorite routes while I'm there. The shaded and swampy Hawthorne Trail in Gainesville, Florida. The rolling country roads through the magnificent horse farms of Kentucky. The endless sand-covered asphalt trails along the Atlantic Ocean in Virginia Beach. Just because there isn't someone waiting for me at the end to drape a medal around my neck doesn't mean it wasn't an amazing experience, because it most certainly was.

Every single one of my runs is rewarding because all of them end exactly the same, and that's what keeps me coming back for more.

I get to cross the finish line. And it doesn't cost me a cent.

Al Barker and I formed the Darkside Running Club in 2002. One of our objectives was to give back to the running community. Another was to return every cent collected through membership dues, entry fees, and the like back to the runners. We're proud to say we've held true to those objectives and will continue to do so in the years ahead.

RUNNING ON FUMES

FEBRUARY 2015

I'm running out of gas.

I know I've said it before, but this time I really, really, really mean it.

I'm literally running out of gas.

I've promised myself more times than I care to admit that I would limit my weekly mileage. It all began in 1998 when I was putting in well over 100 miles a week. Since I wasn't anywhere near world class, had no chance of qualifying for the Olympics, nor earning a living by running lots of miles, I thought it wise to cut back a bit.

A bit. Ninety miles a week for the next eight years hardly qualifies as a bit. So in 2007 I got serious and made a firm commitment to reduce my weekly mileage…to 85 miles a week. OK, baby steps. A few years later (2010) I took it a step further and cut back to 75 a week (more baby steps) where I held steady for a few years.

Then it happened. I turned 60 years old and asked myself as seriously as I'm capable of asking myself a question out loud:

How many 60-year-old men are running 70 miles a week?

(If you happen to know don't tell me because even if it's only one, I'll feel compelled to make it two.)

So now I'm more than five weeks into my 61st year on earth, and I'm still putting in 70 miles a week. But this time I have a reason: My younger son Josh will be running his first marathon soon, and he wants me to run it with him. So I decided to maintain my weekly regimen of 70 miles a week until it got me through Josh's first—and my last—marathon on the 15th of February.

Let me back up for a moment. I'll admit I ran my "last" marathon in Honolulu a couple of years ago during the weekend I turned 58. I'll also admit there were three other "last" marathons after that. But this time—once (if) I cross the finish line of the Five Points of Life Marathon in Gainesville, Florida—it will effectively signal the end of my marathon career. That's all, folks; color me done.

Coincidentally I ran my very first marathon in that same city—Gainesville—a little more than six years before Josh was born. I was wearing my $5 USA Olympic size 9 running shoes that I bought from the original Athletic Attic which was located about three miles from the trailer park I lived in during my senior year at the University of Florida. (Today I wear a size 10, the larger feet no doubt a result of the millions of times they slapped the asphalt over the years.)

This marathon will be special for three reasons. The first two are obvious: It will be Josh's first and my last. The third reason is I'll be promoting an insole company I represent all over the world—all over the world that isn't the United States, that is—on American soil. I'll be wearing the company's singlet that arrived in the mail the other day. While it fits perfectly and is made of a fabric I like, it has the most hideous color scheme you'd ever want to run across. At the top of the singlet the color is sort of a faded coral, and as you work your way down the singlet the color morphs through various colors until you reach the very bottom of the singlet where there is a color best described as dry urine.

Speaking of dry urine (also known as the official color of done)…

That's an apt description of how I've been feeling lately. I've had some sort of flu off and-on (mostly on) for the past five weeks. In fact I've been sick more days this year alone than in all the years I've been running combined. I'm thinking my immune system is waving the white flag. Various parts of my body ache almost every day; I imagine they're rebelling because they haven't had any real down time since 1978. I yawn all the time, the result of a lifetime of sleep deprivation that began with the birth of my first son in 1982. That was the year I started to run in the morning, and with a job that required me to be at work as early as 5 a.m., well… feel free to do the math.

So I'm still putting in 70 miles a week until I get through this next/last marathon. After that I'm cutting back.

I really, really, really mean it this time.

Really.

Postscript: They day after I wrote this I ran 10 miles and then another mile in a fun-run with my grandson. The next day I ran 15 miles with Josh, our last long run before the marathon—then only a week away. I made plans to take it easy up until and then after the marathon. After that, I need to be running the mileage expected of a 60-year-old man.

In church the morning after our 15-mile run the pastor said something in his message about asking yourself if you were young or old, and if you had to think about it you were old.

That definitely made me think.

ALL THE PROOF I NEED

FEBRUARY 2015

There was a time when every marathon was an adventure. On race morning I literally couldn't wait to get to the starting line to see what the next 26.2 miles had in store for me. There were old friends, familiar faces, and race directors I knew by name. A plethora of courses I knew like the back of my hand: some easy, some not-so-much, and several somewhere in the middle. Then there was that all too familiar thrill of crossing the finish line just one more time.

Most of all there was the anticipation of what might turn this particular marathon into an adventure. A random stranger asking me at the 10-mile mark if I could get their friend to the finish line in a Boston-qualifying time because the random stranger could no longer keep up the pace; experiencing the effects of consuming a Twinkie and a glass (or two) of champagne at an aid station with 16 miles still left to run; running an entire marathon accompanied by my nine-year-old son…on his bicycle (the fact I had to push him up two mountains did not detract from the experience whatsoever).

But then something strange happened. I was no longer feeling any excitement on the morning of the marathon. Suddenly and without warning the mornings were no longer an adventure. The thrill of finishing…was gone. What changed?

I wasn't seeing the familiar faces I had come to know. Many of my favorite marathons were no more (RIP Atlanta, Tybee Island, Vulcan). Entry fees were increasing at an alarming rate while the quality of the races remained virtually status quo. Marathons simply were no longer any fun.

I had high hopes this would change when I lined up for the Five Points of Life Marathon in Gainesville, Florida. Twenty years after pedaling his two-wheeler beside me for 26.2 miles in Birmingham, Alabama, my son Josh was standing next to me ready, willing, and hopefully able for his first attempt at covering the distance on foot. As for me, this would be my last marathon; the only reason I was running was because I told Josh long ago I would run his first marathon with him. Otherwise my final marathon would have been a little over two years ago (the fact that there have been three others since that time is irrelevant to the fact that Five Points was going to be my final-and-this-time-I-really-really-mean-it final marathon).

So at 7 a.m. on a brisk February morning Josh and I were on our way. We headed north on 34th Street, side by side, stride for stride, and wearing matching Currex Insole singlets. *(Yes, they are a sponsor of mine, and no I don't get paid. Satisfied?)*

Josh had his mind set on running the marathon in 3 hours and 50 minutes. I had my mind set on doing whatever I could to make sure Josh crossed the finish line. We both had our minds set on having a great time.

We both failed. But I take the blame; I should have known better. After all, this wasn't my first rodeo.

Josh was focused on maintaining a pace of 8:40 to 8:50 per mile for as long as he could and then settling for 9-minute miles once fatigue set in. I should have done a better job of having him focus on taking his time, enjoying the experience, and listening to what his body was telling him. Josh's plan worked just fine; that is to say, it worked just fine for the first 18 miles. That's when Josh's legs started to cramp up something fierce.

We took several walk breaks for a couple of miles, then took a couple of running breaks from what essentially had turned into a walk for a couple of miles. Then at the 22-mile aid station Josh laid down on his back and for all intents and purposes his marathon had come to an end. The volunteer—a retired doctor—told Josh his cramps could possibly be the result of dehydration or muscle fatigue and encouraged him to drink lots and lots of Gatorade. Twenty minutes later Josh, still prone on the ground, said he thought he could finish the race. The doctor told him he'd rather see him drop out today and return next year and win than see him continue. The doctor looked at me and said, "*Aren't you his dad? You tell him* [to drop out]!"

Me, the guy who ran practically the entirety of the 100-mile Western States Endurance Run with the balls of his feet split wide open while dismissing the advice of the on-course foot doctor who told him that if he continued (this occurring at mile 62) he could risk infection and the subsequent loss of his feet? *Me*, the guy who ran *(OK, mostly walked. OK, OK, totally walked)* the last 13 miles of the Badwater Ultramarathon bouncing between two members of his support crew so he wouldn't wander off the side of Mount Whitney?

Sorry, doc: You've got the wrong guy. Consider my silence to be your clue.

The doctor said he'd give Josh a ride to the medical station at mile 23. I told him I'd meet them there. I then spent another 10 minutes with Josh at the medical tent—wanting to stay with him on one hand and wanting to get to mile 26 on the other because that is where my wife would be with my grandson who was eager to run the last quarter-mile to the finish line with me.

Once Josh assured me he would be fine, I told him I'd be back for him once I crossed the finish line. The next four miles were torture, the result of my legs tightening up from standing around for the better part of 30 minutes. My grandson Krischan was eager to run when I finally showed up, and believe me when I say it was all I could do to keep up with him for that last 440 yards.

We crossed the finish line together, and I motioned for the finish line volunteer to drape the finisher's medal around Krischan's neck. Krischan, who before today had run four one-mile fun-runs and came to understand that medals are only for those who run in the longer, accompanying 3.1-mile races said, "That didn't *feel* like three miles!"

I then walked to the car and drove back to the 23-mile medical station where Josh said he was given (surprise!) even more Gatorade to drink. He said he felt a little bit better before coming up with this: *"Well, Dad, I guess you're going to have to run one more marathon."*

Postscript: Three days later I received an email with proofs from the race. For those who don't know, proofs are photographs taken of the runners during a race that can set you back about a gazillion dollars. I was surprised to find that there wasn't one single proof of Josh and me running together. Hey race photographers: NEWS FLASH! If you see two runners running side by side, stride by stride in matching singlets who appear to be about a generation apart in age you might want to take a photo with both of them in it as the chances are pretty decent that they might like to have one.

Examining the proofs a little bit more I couldn't help but notice the expression on my face while running with Josh. I'm fishing for a couple adjectives here…let's see. Pained. Exhausted. Old. Yep…old. Sad but true. Josh's face? Stern. Focused. Much, much too serious.

But the proofs with Krischan and me were different. I looked happy. Rested. Young(er), even. In fact, I had the same expression on my face that I remembered from proofs of races I ran in a decade or two ago. A time when I smiled when I was running.

As for Krischan in the photos, it was evident he was just enjoying the moment. He loves to run, and he loves his G-Pa. He didn't know how far we had run, how fast (or slow) we had run, or that I had already run 26 miles before I joined him for the sprint to the finish line. That's how it is when you're enjoying the moment, and that's exactly what I should have passed on to Josh.

There are all kinds of inferences to be made from looking at the photos but one thing is certain: At the moment, I'm not capable of running competitive marathons. The proof is…well, the proof is in the proofs.

I'm sorry Josh didn't finish, but he's young, willing, and one day will be more than capable of running 26.2 miles. If anyone is responsible for Josh not finishing it's me. I knew better, and I should have set a better example. After all, the Five Points of Life Marathon wasn't my first rodeo.

But it may very well be my last.

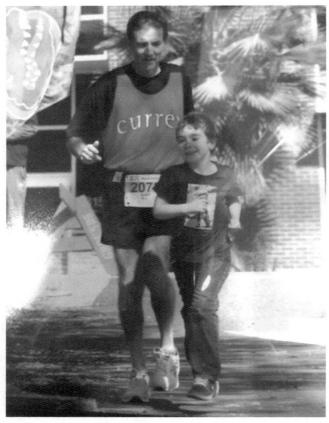

Scott and Krischan at the finish of the Five Points of Life Marathon in Gainesville, Florida

EPIC SH*T

MAY 2015

Today it's referred to as Epic Sh*t. In layman's terms, it means facing your fears, taking calculated risks, and living life to the fullest.

It didn't used to be called that. It used to be called—simply—life.

Here's an example from my younger days:

My entire life I've never been a good swimmer. Imagine my surprise (read: intense trepidation) when I was only 12 years old and required to swim an entire mile as part of a Boy Scout program. Considering that up until then the farthest I had ever swum was one length of the local pool (25 yards), swimming 70 times as far was as close to facing my demons as I ever hope to be. (I also fear heights, being falsely incarcerated, and drinking tequila, but I have no intentions of facing them in this lifetime…or in the case of the tequila, facing *again*.) While I have no memory of how long it took me to swim those 70 lengths of the pool, I remember vividly not being able to pull myself out of the water afterward, my arms rendered worthless after dog paddling for an hour or two (perhaps even three). The bottom line is this: For a 12-year-old boy with limited abilities in all things aquatic, swimming one entire mile was indeed Epic Sh*t…although in 1967 the person who coined the phrase probably hadn't even been born.

My love for running has taken me on quite a few adventures that might fall into the category of Epic Sh*t. Some of them were initially nothing more than Epic Fails, but then again, I've never been particularly good at failure, losing or taking no for an answer, so I gave them a second chance. Consider it to be my character flaw. *(Yes, I have only one if you don't count my total detachment from reality as another.)* Regardless, they all met the Epic Sh*t requirements: I was facing my fears, taking calculated risks, and living life to the fullest.

As for the Epic Fails:

Epic Fail 1: Initial Attempt at Running Across Georgia (280 miles over the course of seven days). On the morning of the fourth day, after three days, four hours, and 159 miles I took out the white flag and surrendered. Actually, it was my legs that surrendered (or perhaps my spirit; can't remember as this happened in 1982). Ten years later I returned to the scene of the crime, only this time I covered all 280 miles. It took six days.

Epic Fail 2: Initial Attempt at the Western States Endurance Run (2004). After 62 miles and 18 hours, with only 38 miles left to run and a generous 12 hours remaining in which to finish, I pulled out the white flag for the second time in my life and called it quits. Again, my legs were responsible (or perhaps my spirit, can't remember as I was comatose within seconds once I officially removed myself from the race). Two years later I returned, completing the 100 miles in a little over 30 hours and finishing in dead last in a race that over half of the field failed to finish for a multitude of reasons, most noticeably the unfavorable conditions encountered on the course (as if 100 miles of mountain trails alone wasn't difficult enough there was snow, melting snow, extreme heat, and dust so thick you could cut if with a knife).

As for Epic Sh*t, I often wonder if I don't do some of the things I do because they make for a good story. Running 135 miles in over 130-degree heat in Death Valley…running 54 miles in South Africa 12 hours after being robbed at knife point…running a marathon in Honolulu with the (Epic Fail) intent of making it my last marathon…starting the Peachtree Road Race from (literally) the back row and passing countless thousands of runners in the 6.2 miles between Atlanta's Lenox Square and Piedmont Park.

If these all qualify as Epic Sh*t, so be it, but that was never the original intent. The intent was simply to prove to myself that I could.

While I have accepted the fact that my days of true Epic Sh*t are behind me, I couldn't help being inspired by the accomplishments of two friends of mine in the past week, making me consider going to the well one more time before calling it a day:

- Joe, who ran an amazing 606 miles in a six-day race in Hungary, beating his closest competitor (literally) by just over 100 miles.

- Dave, who was recognized for his lifetime mileage total reaching a whopping 172,000 miles (and still going strong).

That is indeed some Epic Sh*t.

I realize my days of long, fast(like) runs are behind me. I'm now a full generation removed from sub-2:50 marathons. I'll never finish a 100-mile race again on the same day I started; likely, I'll probably never run another 100-mile race, period. Finishing among the top 1,000 at Peachtree—once a sure bet—is now out of the question, lest there be a complete reversal of fortune with the various ailments affecting my legs and lower back, not to mention my psyche.

Yes, Joe and Dave fascinated me. They also inspired me.

I'm going to do one last run, and I'm going to do it with both guns blazing. It may not be pretty, it may not be fast, and it most definitely won't hold a torch to what Joe and Dave accomplished. But if things go well it could be one last attempt for me to achieve Epic Sh*t.

I just hope it doesn't turn out to be an Epic Dump. Time will tell.

AL AT 70

MAY 19, 2015

Several years ago, Dave, a friend of mine whom I had met at a race in Tennessee over a decade ago, came all the way from Ohio to Peachtree City, Georgia, to compete in one of our Darkside running events. The first thing he asked me the morning of the race was this, *Is Al Barker going to be here?*

Dave had read several of my books and anyone familiar with my publications knows that I spend considerable time writing about the personalities, accomplishments, and idiosyncrasies of my running friends. Of those friends, no one gets more ink (nor has run more miles with me) than Albert E. Barker. It didn't surprise me one bit that Dave would immediately inquire about him on his first venture into Fayette County, Georgia. After all, that's where Al lives. Or rather, where he gained his infamy.

Anyone who has ever read anything I've written about Al over the years—and believe me when I tell you there's a lot to be read—knows four things about him: (1) He's an exceptional runner, (2) he's an exceptional artist, (3) he's an exceptional photographer, and (4) he's an exceptional character. As for the latter, Dave couldn't wait to see the man who snacked on plastic potpourri at a social function because he mistakenly thought they were party snacks…and ate a handful of Starburst candies without removing the wrappers…and poured creamer into his glass of water instead of his coffee, then stirred it up and drank it…and ate an entire order of shrimp with the shells intact because after he ate the first one and his oversight was pointed out he tried to save face by saying that he liked them that way and then had no other choice but to eat every last one of them, shells and all. Dave thought it might be cold enough that Al would show up wearing a cat sweater as he did years ago, thinking he had grabbed his wool cap from the closet before heading out for a run. Dave was anxious to meet the man famous for the quote "Put me down for a turd" and the question "Have you ever stepped in your own sh*t?" *(Let me stop here for a moment: If you want to read more you're just going to have to read my books. No, this isn't a shameless plug: simply a cold, hard fact.)*

Al turns 70 today. It's hard to believe that when we started running together in the fall of 1993 that Al, almost 10 years my senior, was only 48 years old. A lot of time and a lot of miles have accumulated since then. While both of us have slowed down a bit over the years, Al has a lot to be proud of. When he was 50 years old he ran a marathon in St. George, Utah, a few seconds over three hours. When he was 60 years old he ran 100 miles in San Diego, California, in less than 24 hours. In his 50s he earned a piece of two Guinness World Records as a member of both the men's masters and grandmasters 100 x 1-mile relay teams.

Before I met Al, he had run a sub-five-minute mile and a Boston Marathon in the low 2:50s, not to mention numerous 10Ks in the 35- to 36-minute range. The man had speed, endurance, and a finishing kick that ranks with the best of them. He still has the latter, in fact. Do you know the joke about the two runners trying to elude a bear and one runner says to the other "we have to outrun this bear or we're both going to die," and the other runner says "no, I just have to outrun *you*"? I mention it because if Al and I are ever running together near his cabin in the mountains of North Carolina and a bear comes chasing after us, Al will soon be busy writing my eulogy.

Al has already had quite an exciting year in 2015. Last month he became a grandfather for the first time. Al's daughter Ashley and her husband Cameron became the proud parents of twin daughters Emery and Conner. Al's first question to me after telling me the news of the latest addition to the Barker clan was "How old were you when you ran your first race with Krischan?" It didn't surprise me one bit, because I know how anxious he is to share the things that mean the most to him with the people he loves. And Al certainly loves his granddaughters. *(Be ready, girls: Paint brushes and cameras won't be too far behind your first pair of running shoes!)*

As you might have guessed Al still has his competitive spirit. Next month Al and I are running in a 5K race—a race he served as race director in its first year over three decades ago—as he is eager to see how he will fare in his new age group. I remember a while back—about the time he turned 60, I believe—Al could tell who was in his age group by the number of wrinkles on the back of his competitors' necks. Something tells me that when he runs in that first 5K in his new age group he won't be seeing too many wrinkled 70-year-old necks in front of him. The man can still run.

Getting back to Dave from Ohio and wanting to meet Al, I'm happy to report that the two of them did meet that day and hit it off immediately. Although Al wasn't running in the race, he was going to lead the first 5.2-mile loop of the race on his bicycle. A couple of minutes after I gave the "Go" command to start the race, I saw Al walking back toward the starting line, guiding his bicycle with one hand and a shoe in the grasp of the other. It seems Al's shoe was untied and the lace got tangled in the bicycle chain, forcing the tires to come to a sudden stop and causing Al to fly over the top of the handlebars and onto the ground in full view of all the runners.

It's safe to assume Dave got what he came to Georgia looking for.

THE NEXT BIG THING

JUNE 2015

"You wouldn't understand."

Those are the only words that came to mind when my wife asked me why…probably because I wasn't sure I understood it myself. She asked again. This time I upgraded my answer to "I just have to."

Cindy has known me since I was 18 years old. By now she knows me well enough to know that sometimes "I just have to" is the only explanation I can offer.

I've been a runner for a long time. Certainly long enough to know when it's time to take a step back from anything that could have adverse effects on my health and safety, such as

- running across Death Valley in the hottest part of the summer;

- running 280 miles across the width of Georgia;

- celebrating my 60th birthday by running 60 miles, then shortly afterward running 60 kilometers as a cool-down;

- running a marathon not long after running what I said would be my last one, which was then followed by the one after that and the one after that; or

- the same thing after running what I said would be my last ultra-marathon. It wasn't. I ran another, then one more after that.

Those days have come and gone. Almost.

Thinking back over anything and everything I've ever tried in my running career, they all have one thing in common: I did them because I had it in my mind that I just had to. Meanwhile Cindy was always nervously anticipating my next big thing and knowing that—whatever it was—she didn't have a prayer of talking me out of it.

But now I'm at the point where I realize that continuing to do things of this nature just doesn't make any sense.

Which is precisely the reason I came up with this: The Last Big Thing.

This is the one that I know in my heart will be *the* last one. This Next Big Thing will certainly be my last. I've been thinking about this one ever since the idea came to me, and I've totally convinced myself this will turn out to be "the one." After this I won't have a reason to try anything else, if for no other reason than this one is going to get everything I've got. After this—if all goes as planned—there won't be anything left for me to give.

I'm calling it the Senoia 60, and this is how it works: I want to run as far as I can in the 60 hours between 6 a.m. Friday, October 23, and 6 p.m. Sunday, October 25. The eight-mile route will start and finish in Haralson, Georgia, but most of the loop that will be used for the event is actually in neighboring Senoia. There will be one central aid station (which will also be used for parking) close to the spot where (SPOILER ALERT) Daryl Dixon killed his brother-turned-zombie Merle on *The Walking Dead*.

Now for the really fun part: The event is open to the public! The more the merrier. After all, misery loves company, and if things go as planned I can be assured of my fair share. The slogan for the weekend is "Run to the Edge" and was chosen with one thought in mind: I've been running and pushing myself to the edge of exhaustion for as long as I care to remember. This is my chance to do the very thing I've always professed to be doing all along. I simply want to discover what my breaking point is…the exact moment when I've literally fallen over the edge into true, unadulterated exhaustion. I just hope I'm coherent enough to recognize it when it happens; if not I'm hoping the other runners (Remember: Misery loves company. Lots of it.) will be able to assist.

I don't know what those 60 hours have in store for me, but this I can be sure of: Win, lose or crawl it will certainly be my Last Big Thing.

In all honesty, it is the one remaining thing I need to do before I will be free of having to do anything else simply because I just have to.

If none of this makes any sense to you, then you simply wouldn't understand.

TAKING CARE OF BUSINESS

JUNE 2015

In the fall of 1993, Al, Val, and I were running 20 miles religiously every Sunday. There were exceptions, of course. Three to be exact: running a marathon, running an ultra, or death. Other than that, we all knew the drill, a drill we would continue well into the next century.

Val and I ran the 1993 Atlanta Marathon together stride for stride and fast enough for her to qualify for her first Boston Marathon. Al met us at the finish line, and the two of them agreed they would be in Beantown the following April and wanted me to be there as well. There was only one problem: I did not have a Boston qualifying time and up until that moment was perfectly content with my one Boston Marathon—a PR, by the way so why jeopardize that kind of karma?—back in 1987.

But they insisted on me being with them for Val's first—and Al's third—Boston Marathon. They immediately began looking at race calendars to find a possible marathon for me to run a qualifying time. It wasn't long before all of us were signed up for the 1994 Tallahassee Marathon: our first business trip marathon.

The ideal business trip marathon is completed within 24 hours. Here's how Tallahassee played out:

- Pack a bag with running gear and place in trunk of car on

Friday morning. (This is considered prep time; at this point the 24-hour clock hasn't started.)

- Friday, 6:00 p.m.—Leave for marathon destination after end of work day. (24-hour clock begins.)

- Friday, 11:00 p.m.—Check into hotel; spend the night.

- Saturday, 5:30 a.m.—Wake up. Eat breakfast at hotel (optional, and only if complementary).

- Saturday, 7:00 a.m.—Run marathon.

- Saturday, 11:00 a.m.—Return to hotel. Shower (ask hotel staff for late checkout if needed).

- Saturday, 12:00 p.m.—Drive home.

- Saturday, 5:00 p.m.—Arrive home. (Mission accomplished; elapsed time of 23 hours.)

I would be remiss in telling about our first official business trip marathon if I failed to mention our hotel accommodations. I won't mention the hotel by name, but I will tell you (a) it was not part of a chain, (b) there was a life-size white ceramic Brahman bull in front of the hotel, and (c) the towels in the rooms were so old and worn you could (literally) see through them. Anyway, Al and I shared a room, and Val had a room to herself. The hotel manager agreed to let us have a late checkout, but only in one of the rooms. After the marathon Al and I quickly grabbed our bags and a couple of towels from our room as the three of us had decided to take turns showering in Val's room, the one with the late checkout.

When we went into the lobby to pay the hotel manager tried to charge Al and me for two towels as the maid had already reported them missing from our room.

Getting back to the story...

Two months later the three of us made the trip to Boston and would go on to run many more marathons in the years ahead, most of them of the business-trip variety.

This past weekend was the first time Al and I ever took a Business Trip 5K. But this was no regular 5K: This was the 37th running of the Kiwanis Melon Run 5K in Monticello, Florida. Al just so happened to be the race director the first year the race was held in 1979. But this particular edition of the event had a special affinity for Al: It was the first race he could run as a 70-year-old. As for me, it was sort of a cosmic calling to return to the area where we ran our first business trip marathon over 20 years ago (Monticello is about 30 miles from Tallahassee). Contrary to what some people might think, the fact I was now a 60-year-old and in a new age group as well had nothing to do with my decision to tag along. (In other news, I'm prone to lie to embellish a story.)

Here's how our first official Business Trip 5K turned out:

• Friday, 5:30 p.m.: Leave for Monticello after end of workday. (24-hour clock begins.)

• Friday, 11:00 p.m.: Check into hotel. Turn on air conditioner in room because it's easily 120 degrees in a room that's been baking in the 100-degree sun all day long.

- Saturday, 5:15 a.m.: Wake up. Take quick showers after six hours of sleeping in a sauna. Eat complimentary breakfast in hotel lobby approximately the size of a walk-in closet (the lobby, not the breakfast) under the watchful eye of the front desk clerk who makes sure none of the guests take more than one muffin or yogurt cup. (I took one of each; I was asked never to return.)

- Saturday, 7:00 a.m.: Arrive at race site; pick up race number. Run the course as a warm-up; make mental note that this could possibly turn out to be the toughest 3.1-mile route I've ever run.

- Saturday, 8:00 a.m.: Find unattended restroom; make mental note what a stroke of luck the restroom remained unattended the entire time I was inside. (TMI? Perhaps.)

- Saturday, 8:15 a.m.: Race begins. Course takes a 90-degree right turn after only 80 meters; I note two runners—a husband and wife—both pushing baby strollers are ahead of me. I curse silently to myself.

- Saturday, 8:22:15 a.m.: One mile down. Just like that— *BOOM!* I am now in front of the baby stroller being pushed by the dad. Mom will be next. I haven't seen Al since the race began; I wonder how he's doing.

- Saturday, 8:30:20: Two miles down. The course is beautiful; I already look like crap (the race photos I receive later will prove me correct). Mom with baby stroller is nowhere in sight. I look back over my shoulder and notice the same thing about Al.

- Saturday, 8:something: I have 400 meters to the finish line: Every one of them is *straight up a hill!* I doubt my ability to continue running to the finish line and wonder if this will be the first 5K I fail to run the entire way.

- Saturday, 8:something: I cross the finish line, proud of myself for running the entire way but disappointed with my finishing time. However, the relief of finishing the most difficult 5K course I've ever run overshadows the aforementioned disappointment.

- Saturday, 8:something but pretty darn close to 9:00 a.m.: Al is navigating his way up the 400 meters to the finish. I can only imagine what his race photos will look like, but it's a pretty safe bet he won't want to see them. (Later I am again proven correct.)

- Saturday, 10:30 a.m.: Awards ceremony. All age-group winners receive a medal and a watermelon; second and third place in each five-year age group receive a medal. I won third place in my age group and receive a medal for my 20-something minutes of work; Al finishes fourth in his age group, and his former dentist who is volunteering at the race gives him a Monticello Watermelon Festival baseball cap. I'd much rather have the baseball cap than the medal.

- Saturday, 11:00 a.m.: Towel dry, change clothes, and head home.

- Saturday, 3:45 p.m.: Arrive home. (Mission accomplished; elapsed time of 22 hours and 15 minutes.)

Now that the dust has settled and I look back on our first Business Trip 5K, it made me think back to the times when we were traveling to run races that took more than one day to complete. That was followed by a subsequent step down to traveling only to races we could finish in the same day they began.

This weekend we traveled to a race we could finish in the same hour it began.

Even if it was only by the skin of Al's teeth…

BABY, THE RAIN MUST FALL

JULY 4, 2015

I run for many reasons. It's good for the body, mind, and soul. It allows me to eat an extra dessert (or two) relatively guilt-free. It makes me feel good (*most of the time, anyway*). It gives me a pair of legs to die for (*discuss quietly among yourselves*).

In other words, it's no secret I love running.

It's also no secret I've done a lot of the things I've done simply because I made them a goal, and I did whatever it took to make them happen:

- Running a mile without stopping.

- Running a 10K without stopping.

- Qualifying for the Boston Marathon.

- Running the Boston Marathon.

It's also no secret I've done a lot of the things I've done simply because they seemed like a good idea at the time:

- Running 135 miles across Death Valley in temperatures very, very close to the number of miles.

- Entering the Western States Endurance Run—twice, actually—when I had absolutely no business running on trails. (If Montrail named a shoe after me it would be the Nontrail. If New Balance named a shoe after me it would be the No Balance. Any questions?)

It's also no secret I've done a lot of the things I've done simply because it gave me something interesting to write about:

- Running the Boston Marathon course in reverse, then turning around and running it the correct way with everyone else on Patriot's Day.

- Running the Peachtree Road Race from the very back of the pack. In other words, starting behind 59,999 other runners for a 6.2-mile run on the Fourth of July in downtown Atlanta.

Finally, it's no secret I do a lot of the things I do simply because. In other words, I'm prone to putting requirements on myself that no one in the solar system gives a rat's a** about other than yours truly. Such as:

- Running every day since November 30, 1978 (with no end in sight).

- Running 1,000 races, 200 marathons, and 50 ultras (two down, one to go).

- Running 150,000 lifetime miles (ETA 2018).

- Running 50 consecutive Peachtree Road Races (ETA 2028).

Ah, that last one. Fifty consecutive Peachtree Road Races. Having just crossed the finish line for the 37th time, I'm beginning to question if I still have 13 more of them in me. Allow me to explain.

The Peachtree Road Race assigns runners a starting corral. My finish time in last year's Peachtree qualified me for a spot in Time Group A, which basically means you are assigned to a corral close enough to the starting line that you can read the word "START" on the banner across Peachtree Street and in all probability will finish the race in well under an hour. (Time Groups B through L will finish the race in less than two hours, M through V in less than three hours, and W through Z sometime during the month of July. I jest, of course. Almost everyone in W through Z time groups finish in time to see the fireworks later that same night.)

Anyway, I opted to start in Time Group L with my friend Valerie who submitted her application for the race without a projected finish time and was at the mercy of the Atlanta Track Club's method of random Time Group assignment. Valerie and I ran our first Peachtree together in 1994. Incidentally after that race it rained for two days (the result of tropical storm Alberto) in the Atlanta area, causing floods that resulted in considerable damage and the loss of 30 lives.

As we were driving to the race there was an interview with a former director of the Peachtree Road Race on the radio. As the skies overhead became darker and darker I heard her say that the chances of lightning in Atlanta in the morning were pretty slim because most of the storms in the area occurred in the afternoon. I couldn't help but think those words should not have been said aloud, especially in a forum that could be heard by many. Moments later the rain came; it wouldn't stop for hours. For the first time in my Peachtree Road Race career I would be running from Lenox Square to Piedmont Park in the rain that, to be totally honest, was a lot more pleasurable than the usual heat and 100% humidity we've all come to know and abhor.

As I've done for the past decade, we parked near the finish line and ran to the start. Taking the back roads Valerie and I ran (and occasionally walked) a slow and easy five-mile warm up. Wearing my Time Group A number, I stood out like a sore thumb standing next to Val in Time Group L. Actually, I stood out like a STUD— remember, I was amongst runners who hoped to finish in modest times in the one- to two-hour range and my number indicated I was a STUD. (*Pardon my use of Exaggeration Font. I don't get to use it often.*)

Every three minutes another wave of runners could start the race. Every three minutes volunteers led the runners in Time Group L another 100 yards closer to the starting line. Every three minutes the sky grew darker and darker. The race officially started at 7:30 a.m. By my calculation Time Group L's projected starting time would be around 8:30.

Then, at 8:24 a.m., it happened. A bolt of lightning flashed across the sky. The announcer on the PA system immediately said the race had been suspended, the timing system would be stopped, everyone would be led to safe quarters, and the race would resume in 30 minutes unless more lightning was spotted. Surely he realized there were thousands of runners spread out all over Peachtree Street; did he expect everyone to stop, mark their spot on the course, and seek shelter?

Val and I looked around, and we knew what had to be done. Others had the same idea as well. In a driving rain and with the wind in our collective faces, we all took off running down Peachtree Street like bats out of hell, timing system be damned. We were running this race come hell or (*forgive me*) high water. As far as we were concerned Time Group L had heard a public cry for a jailbreak over the public-address system. From what I saw the same can be said for Time Groups J, K, and M. I'm guessing Time Groups N through Z heard it as well. There would be very little need for the safe quarters that the announcer had made reference to. Not today anyway, because today we were here to run.

As Val and I left Lenox Square behind us, I couldn't help but notice that had I started with Time Group A moments after 7:30 a.m. I would have already crossed the finish line. As it was, it was already 8:30, and I was just starting the race, and as far as I knew I wasn't even an official runner since the timing system had allegedly been stopped. I wondered if my streak of Peachtree Road Race finishes was in jeopardy, but I didn't care: I was not going to wait in the pouring rain for 30 minutes, resume my position with Time Group L, and continue the 100-yards-every-three-minutes march toward the starting line.

As it turned out the 6.2 miles down Peachtree Street was quite pleasant. The steady rain and gentle breeze kept the runners cool as well as hydrated. Val had (what she said afterward was) her best run in years. We crossed the finish line in a little over an hour, collected our commemorative finisher T-shirts, and headed back to the car. As we made our way across the grass of Piedmont Park I couldn't help but think of the famous 1969 Woodstock music festival: There was mud everywhere. The rain and the runners were certainly taking their toll on this most unusual Fourth of July.

Once we got back to the car we changed into dry clothes. I placed my running attire in a plastic bag and tied it shut, making a mental note to throw all the contents into the washing machine once I got home. *(Runners—you all know the drill: Wash the clothes today or burn them tomorrow.)*

Overall this year's Peachtree Road Race was a good experience, with the exceptions of paying $15 to park for 15 minutes so you can run into the expo to pick up your race number and a goodie bag featuring nothing more than a coupon for a free waffle, a $500 discount on a new Mercedes Benz, and a plethora of advertisements.

My 37th Peachtree Road Race finish was in the books.

Maybe.

(Later I would learn the timing system had never been turned off. Valerie and I both received official finishing times.
 Next year Valerie hopes to qualify for a starting position in Time Group B, if not A.

Fortunately for me I will still be eligible for Time Group A.

After next year I may find myself at the mercy of the Gods of Random Time Group Assignment.

If that's the case, then God help me.

TRAIL RUNNING. YAY!

JULY 2015

There. I've done it again.

In this particular case "it" would be running on trails and "again" a reference to falling. For me the two go hand in hand.

Or in my particular case: Body to ground.

After this last fall, if you ever see me running on trails (and after this latest escapade the chances of that are beyond miniscule) feel free to mock, ridicule, or shame me—whatever you feel is appropriate. But first, let me explain what happened.

Cindy and I were in Colorado Springs for a weekend getaway. After a miserable experience running on the streets, exit ramps, and frontage roads the first day, I noticed several runners on a dirt path about a quarter-mile from our hotel as I began my run on the second day. The trail was fairly smooth, generously wide, and virtually free of the rocks and sticks found on most of the trails I've run in the southeast.

"Why not?" I thought. "I could use a run without having to dodge traffic, jump on and off curbs, and worrying about an SUV slamming in to me after blowing out a tire at 70 miles per hour." Don't laugh: An SUV did exactly that the day before, except instead of veering off to the right side of the road where I was running it veered to the left and scraped against an iron guard rail for 100 yards or so. I took that as a sign to avoid the busy roads if there was any way possible. This newfound trail made it possible…

…and falling on a gritty dirt trail was a lot better option than being struck from behind by an out-of-control SUV moving at 70 miles per hour.

And falling is exactly what I did less than two miles into my planned 10-mile Sunday morning run. I didn't fall on my own; I had help. A boulder the size of a running shoe (of course some may consider it a pebble) jumped out in front of me and caused me to trip. (The pebble…I mean boulder…may have been imbedded in the ground; the memories in my head are cloudy at best.) I landed squarely on the palms of my hands, my chest, my hips, and my left knee. I slid face-down on the ground for a couple of feet (the umpire at second base called me safe), came to a halt, rolled over on my back, and shouted out an artisan word or three. The first thought that crossed my mind was "Damn, my hands hurt; I wonder if I'll be able to type." Note the thought of not being able to run never crossed my mind. I didn't move a muscle for a good three or four minutes, wondering how much damage I had done to my body this time. I say, "this time" because as you may have already surmised this wasn't my first time around the block.

Two runners saw me lying prone on the ground and stopped to ask me if I was OK. "Yes," I said. I lied. Both of the palms of my hands were torn open, bleeding profusely, and as I found out a little over eight miles later (You didn't think I wasn't going to finish my run, did you?), full of dirt and grit. Trail shrapnel, I call it. A circle of skin about three inches in diameter was torn from my left kneecap. There was a patch of road rash on my left hip about three times as large as the hole in my knee. I was covered in trail dust and sweat, looking for a place to wash off the dirt and blood. I couldn't find any access to the stream running parallel to the trail so I wore my cloak of crud for a little over an hour before I could get back to the hotel room and jump in the shower. I was running a pretty good pace, hoping I could get my mileage in before I ran out of blood. (I did. The former, not the latter.)

By the time I finished my run the blood had saturated the sock on my left foot. I walked through the hotel lobby, praying that no one eating the breakfast buffet would see me lest I ruin their appetite. Then again, if they did see me, it might mean more food for me later so it's not like I had someone push me through the lobby in a laundry hamper or anything.

So once I got back to our room on the fourth floor, anxious to clean myself up and assess the bodily damage, Cindy is in the shower and guess who no longer has the card key to the room that was safely tucked in his running shorts before taking a nose dive on the trail? So I waited and watched as the blood finally started to dry. I looked at the palms of my hands, unable to distinguish between bruise, blood, and shrapnel. "This can't be good," I thought to myself. I have to admit, I can be sharp as a tack at times.

Once Cindy was out of the shower and let me in the room (when she saw me she didn't flinch; this wasn't her first time around the block either), I jumped in the shower. But not before I went into my ohh-God-it-hurts-so-much-I-think-I'm-going-to-die routine, which had no impact whatsoever when she asked me how many miles I ran…after falling.

As for the shower, let's just say the pain I felt once the water hit my skin made the pain I felt when I first hit the trail feel like a slap on the wrist. Cindy didn't hear my blood-curdling screams because she couldn't hear them over her blow dryer. Probably a good thing, though; I doubt the screams would have gotten me much sympathy. I used a wash rag to scour my hands, trying my best to get rid of as much shrapnel as I could. As hard as I scrubbed, I'm certain I will always have a part of Colorado with me.

The next morning I went out for my last run before heading to the airport for our flight home. I ran on the roads for a while, but once I had dodged enough cars for one day I went back to the trail for those last couple of miles. I ran without incident—a rarity for me on the trails to be sure—the only exception being a brief moment to stop and pay my respects to the boulder (rock; tomato/tomato) that tripped me up 24 hours earlier.

Pay my respects. Feel free to interpret that any way you like. Just know it was my way of saying goodbye to trail running forever.

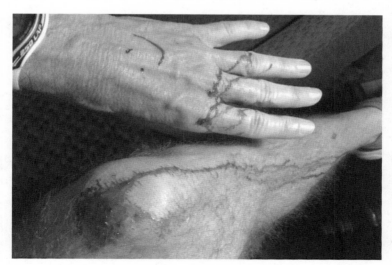

Evidence of Scott having no business running trails ever again

LEGENDARY LUNCH

JULY 2015

My wife Cindy and I had the opportunity to knock two things off our mutual Bucket List not long ago when we discovered Neil Young was going to be in concert at the Red Rocks Amphitheater in Morrison, Colorado. Once we found out it wasn't long before flights were booked, reservations were made, and concert tickets were purchased. It was our first truly spontaneous vacation in all the years we've been married.

We stayed in a hotel in Evergreen the first night, about a 15-minute drive from the amphitheater. Both the concert and the venue were magnificent and well worth the time and money spent. The day after the concert we had the pleasure of having lunch with two of the more notable people in the world of endurance running: Marshall Ulrich and his lovely wife, Heather. Marshall's main claim to fame—although trust me when I tell you it's only the tip of the iceberg—is his double-digit finishes in the Badwater Ultramarathon. Heather's name became somewhat of a household word when she rose to prominence as Marshall's crew chief, support, and go-to person during his 52-day, 3,063-mile run across the United States in 2008 (an adventure chronicled in a book as well as a movie). Believe me when I tell you the four of us had a lot to talk about.

Marshall spoke about some of his more memorable adventures (for the life of me I don't know how he was able to pare his extensive athletic résumé down to a half-dozen items or so) and some of the people in the world of endurance athletics that he admires before transitioning to questioning me about *my* running. (While my experiences in the sport pale in comparison to Marshall's, I will have you know that we've shared many of the same physical as well as psychological ailments over the years. So we're much more alike than you might imagine.) Marshall also mentioned that the wear and tear of his run across the country, now almost seven years ago, took a much bigger toll on Heather than it did on him.

Heather spoke about her experiences being there for Marshall through the years in his quest to test his limits. In fact, she gave up a rewarding full-time job so she could support her husband's interests. She spoke of wanting to be there to support Marshall and that when he was hurting, so was she. While not actively participating in the event per se, she knew exactly what her husband was going through. In other words, it was a challenge being in love with a person who willingly subjected himself on a regular basis to the most demanding physical and psychological challenges imaginable…just to see what he was capable of. Cindy mentioned that she completely understood; after all, she married someone with the same mindset as Marshall's.

We spent almost two hours reliving the past, dreaming of the future, and talking about how much Colorado—the Ulrichs' home— had to offer. Marshall mentioned how they had recently moved from Idaho Springs to Evergreen. They had been living at 10,000 feet elevation, and the extreme altitude was making his running more and more difficult. (Evergreen was at slightly over 7,000 feet elevation, and after my breathtaking—and I don't mean that in a good way—run earlier in the day I couldn't imagine how difficult running at 10,000 feet would be. I don't want to find out, either.)

Our first 24 hours in Colorado were absolutely amazing. Cindy and I crossed two things off our Bucket List, and we got to spend some time with perhaps the most notable couple in the world of endurance running. I also wondered how much pain and suffering I've inflicted on Cindy over our years together as I crossed one thing after another off on my personal Bucket List of Running. I thought about how much she'd been with me, literally and figuratively every step of the way.

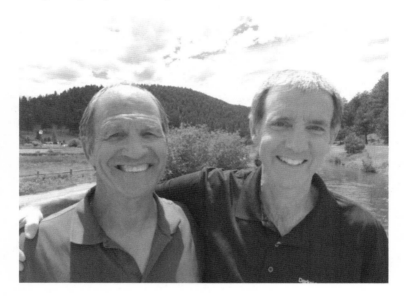

Scott and Marshall Ulrich in Evergreen, Colorado

After lunch we all walked over to Evergreen Lake to take photos of Marshall and me for a forthcoming book* I'm authoring and that Marshall is featured in. Cindy and Heather placed us in several spots for just the right picture. I asked for a shot of the four of us, but the wives insisted the photo should simply be Marshall and me.

---

* *Note: The book,* Running to Extremes: The Legendary Athletes of Ultrarunning, *was published in 2016.*

It was at that moment it dawned on me that I had just eaten lunch with two of the true legends in the sport of long-distance running. Two people, the likes of whom the sport wouldn't be the same without.

Marshall is pretty special, too.

EXTREMES SACRIFICE

AUGUST 2015

The finishing touches were just made on my latest book project, *Running to Extremes: The Legendary Athletes of Ultrarunning.* The book, scheduled for publication by Meyer & Meyer Sport in the spring of 2016 portrays 15 fascinating people in the sport of long-distance running. The project was so vast I couldn't possibly have done it alone. So I asked a few friends—and accomplished runners—if they'd mind joining me. To their credit, they all said yes.

Therefore, I want to recognize those who sacrificed their time and effort towards the publication of the book. Each of these contributors—all more than worthy of being written about in books themselves—has helped make the compilation of the book an exciting and pleasurable experience for me. I also thought it might be a good time to whet your appetite towards reading it someday.

Ladies and gentlemen, my fantastic writing staff:

Steve Boone. Steve lives and runs in Humble, Texas. He has over 600 marathon finishes to his credit that include a marathon in all 50 states five times and more than 200 in the state of Texas. He co-founded the 50 States Marathon Club with his wife Paula in 2001 which now boasts a membership of 3,700. He started and continues to fund the Marathon Challenge Program, which awards T-shirts to local elementary school children who complete the marathon distance during the academic school year.

Over the last 22 years the program has grown from 14 finishers the first year to 9,300 finishers in 2014. Steve and Paula traveled to Kochi, India, in 2014 to start the program in their local elementary schools.

Bonnie Busch. Born, raised, and still living in Iowa, Bonnie has been doing information technology work for over 25 years for an equipment manufacturer. She started recreational running in 1982 to complete the Bix 7-Mile Road Race with a group of friends. She "accidentally" discovered ultrarunning six years later through a local 24-hour run and slowly started to discover ultrarunning events from 50K to multiday adventures on both roads and trails. Among her credentials are 40-plus races of 100 miles or more, 190-plus ultramarathon finishes, the 1995 National USA 24-Hour Female Championship, three Badwater finishes, a solo run across Iowa, and learning how to swim in 2005 and going on to complete 15 Ironman events. Bonnie is still running and willing to try anything once.

Gary Corbitt. Gary is retired from a 38-year career in Media Research. Today he focuses his attention on preserving the history of long-distance running. As curator of the Ted Corbitt Archives his primary mission is preserving his father's legacy and that of the other Founding Fathers of Long-Distance Running.

Gary had a unique view of watching the sport being invented. He considers himself a historian of the sport and remembers when women couldn't officially run in road races or race in track meets at distances farther than 800 meters. As a child and teenager, Gary often volunteered in various capacities at races. He been a fan of the sport since the early 1960s and continues to run races today in the 60 to 64 age category.

David Corfman. David began running marathons in 1997, and four years later he began adding ultramarathons to his résumé. Today he has over 60 finishes in both. His running accomplishments include a silver buckle at Western States in 2009, a Badwater finish in 2010, and 1,000-mile buckles at both the Mohican 100-Mile Trail Race and the Potawatomi Trail Race. He currently leads pace groups at marathons and directs the Stone Steps 50K Trail Race in Cincinnati while continuing to race long distances. David's favorite race distance is 100 miles, where he has painfully learned that no finish is ever given or assumed, and every finish is a triumph.

Dave Dial. Dave grew up in rural east Texas and had a horse before he ever had a bicycle. However, he is fond of saying he found his legs first. With that in mind, it was as a child he initially discovered his love for running. By his teen years, having already run numerous miles on dirt roads and through forest trails in the Davy Crockett National Forest—to get from one place to another or simply for fun—he began keeping a running log in a spiral notebook. Some 40-odd years later Dave currently works as a cattle ranch foreman on land owned by his family for decades. As for running, he has amassed over 171,000 lifetime miles. He also serves as an ambassador for Injinji Footwear and tests high-performance athletic shoes for Sketchers.

Mark Falcone. Mark is retired after 30 years working in the field of technology. He met Tim Twietmeyer 16 years ago when the two of them stopped working for Corporate America and ventured into their own startup. Mark and Tim run, ride, and serve as long-term board members of the Western States Endurance Run Foundation. They both share a love for the preservation of trails.

David Horton. David is a professor of Exercise Science at Liberty University (Lynchburg, Virginia). He currently directs three ultramarathons: Holiday Lake 50K, Promise Land 50K, and Hellgate 100K. David ran for 33 years, compiling over 113,000 miles and 160 ultramarathons. He set speed records for the 2,144-mile Appalachian Trail in 1991 and the 2,650-mile Pacific Crest Trail in 2005. After injuring his knee in 2010 (requiring a total knee replacement in 2014) David converted to ultradistance mountain biking and has completed the 2,700-mile Tour Divide (2011) and has plans to do it again in the near future.

Ben Jones. Ben, a three-time finisher of the Badwater Ultramarathon, was inducted into the Badwater Hall of Fame in 2010. The Mayor of Badwater (as Ben is known) and his wife Denise (the First Lady, who was also inducted) were recognized for their years of service on the race course as athletes, camp hosts, volunteers, crew members, and race ambassadors. Denise has crewed for Ben three times at Badwater and has this to say about him: "He is delightful to his crew, is one of the best-natured people on the planet, never complains, and is always kind. Crewing was always fun."

Norm Klein. Norm and his wife Helen served as co-race directors for 100 races of marathon distance or longer, including the prestigious Western States Endurance Run for 14 years (1986-1999) and the Helen Klein ultra events for 16 years (1995-2010). Norm, an athlete himself, completed over 40 marathons, 40 ultramarathons, an Ironman (Hawaii), and a 125-mile staged race in the Himalayas. In May of 2017 Norm and Helen celebrated their 50th wedding anniversary.

Susan Paraska. Susan ran her first race (a 5K) on July 4, 1986, in Montgomery, Alabama. While living in Colorado in the 1990s she began running 10Ks. After moving to Atlanta, Georgia, she discovered a robust and rich running community offering year-round running at every distance. She completed her first ultra in 2008 (Peachtree City 50K) and her first 100-mile run four years later at the Bartram 100 in Milledgeville, Georgia. Susan is an active member of the Galloway Program and the Darkside Running Club. She is a retired military officer and a certified project manager currently living in Marietta, Georgia.

Chris Roman. Chris is 46 years young and is a doctor, husband, father, philanthropist, and ultrarunner (although not necessarily in that order). In 2004 he decided to get his health back and began training for a marathon that he would eventually complete in slightly less than four hours. Four years later he ran his first 100-mile race in Leadville, Colorado. Since then he has completed some of the more challenging races on the planet including Badwater (twice) and the Brazil 135 (four times). Chris also holds the American Course record on both the 135-mile and 175-mile courses of the Brazil 135. At this time, he is the only person to have run the length of the Eric Canal (344 miles in a little over six days) and one of three people to successfully run Brazil's *Camniho da Fe* (Path of Faith) which he did in just over seven days (while completing the Brazil 135 along the way). Since 2008 Chris has finished 25 races of 100 miles or more. He says the best part is that he has fun every step and now has two distinct families that care for him as much as he cares for them.

Erin Roman. Forever student, teacher, designer, mother, seeker; Erin's passions run deep. As a committed student and teacher of yoga, Erin has been a dedicated practitioner for over 10 years. Mother of two active daughters and wife to her very active husband, her family is her greatest joy and comfort. When she's not running carpool or keeping up with Chris' race schedule she enjoys cooking vegetarian meals for her family, writing blogs, making jewelry, and chasing after their three rescue dogs. In 2014 she expanded her creative reach and opened Carma Blue, her small business "love child." A full plate of family, friends, lesson learning, and big belly laughs her life is perfectly imperfect, and she wouldn't have it any other way.

Erik Schaffer. Erik, a fully certified prosthetist, opened the doors to his own facility, A Step Ahead Prosthetics in Hicksville, New York, in 2001. His philosophy of exacting craftsmanship and innovation and providing a wide variety of prosthetic services under one roof has successfully extended to his business, creating a full ecosystem of support for patients. Erik is considered one of the foremost authorities on prosthetic technology, and A Step Ahead is known as *the* destination for amputees looking for the ultimate in prosthetic care. Erik and his staff were responsible for providing prosthetic care to survivors of the 2013 Boston Marathon bombing.

Craig Snapp. Craig celebrated his 40th year as a runner in 2016 and during that time has never pushed himself to the limits of human endurance, although in recent times he's getting closer to his *own* limits. While not claiming to be an ultrarunner (with only seven runs longer than marathon distance, the longest being 50 miles), he does have a total of 144 marathons and ultramarathons to his credit. One of his memorable moments in running was as a spectator, watching a young Jim Ryun obliterate the high school mile record in 1965 (Ryun ran 3:55.3) which would not be bettered for another 36 years. Having run every single day since April 1, 1998, Craig has managed to accumulate well over 100,000 miles in his running career.

Jon Sutherland. Jon is the current record holder for the longest running streak in America as certified by the USRSA, over 46 years and counting. Jon said, "There is no way I would have ever considered a running streak without my teammate Mark Covert telling me he had run every day for a year. I made a year without missing a day and was fascinated by the journey it took to be a good runner." Jon is an accomplished rock journalist and writer who has been published in over sixty magazines worldwide and has written five books, but his passion has always been running. Jon competed at an international level and raced in many US national championships. Currently Jon is the cross-country coach at Notre Dame High School in Sherman Oaks, California, and enjoys running on the trails behind his house with his dogs Puck and Pixie.

Heather Ulrich. Heather Ulrich was lucky to be born to Rory and Janis Vose and to grow up in Winona, Minnesota, with her two sisters, Laura and Tahra. A bit of a tomboy she went canoeing, camping, hunting, and fishing with her dad, enjoyed horseback riding and Girl Scouts, fell in love with the mountains when working in Yellowstone National Park, and moved permanently to Colorado in the spring of 1990. She met Marshall at the Leadville Trail 100 in 2001 and happily married him on April 1, 2003. (They chose that date because they joked "People will think we're *fools* to be getting married.") While not a runner herself, she enjoys traveling and adventures with Marshall all around the world.

Andy Velazco. Andy started running over 30 years ago while serving in the Army during a hiatus between college and medical school. He has completed over 300 marathons and 70 ultramarathons and after exhaustive research concluded that the best racing distance for him is 50 miles. Andy attributes his best runs to the camaraderie he shares while running with his friends and family.

He takes pride in knowing he introduced his wife and children to running. His wife Kathy has completed 100 marathons, including one in each of the 50 states, and four of his children have two or more marathons under their belts. Andy has run every single Disney World Marathon and has his sights set on being in Orlando for its 25th anniversary in 2018. He has every intention of keeping his passion for running alive in the years ahead.

Marsha White. Marsha ran her first race, a half marathon, at the age of 59 and loved it. Since then she has completed over 200 marathons and ultramarathons in all 50 states, four Canadian provinces, and 10 countries. Now in her late 60s, she frequently places in her age group. Marsha has contributed articles about racing to several books and magazines, including a number of marathon reviews for *Marathon & Beyond*. When she's not traveling to races or writing about them, Marsha enjoys baking, sewing, reading, and quilting.

Amy Yanni. Amy, a self-proclaimed tomboy, has been running all of her life, from softball and tennis to her first race, a five-miler in Northampton, Massachusetts, just before the turn of the century. In 2003, after being diagnosed with breast cancer she started running marathons. Since that time Amy has finished more than 140 marathons, including eight at Boston. She admits she runs a lot simply because she loves to run. Among her many credentials are sub-four-hour marathons in all 50 states after the age of 50 and running a brisk 1:36:03 half marathon at the age of 60 where she edged out Karin Miles, who competed in the Olympic Trials with Joanie Benoit.

Vikena Yutz. Vikena has been running since 2007, and it didn't take her long to fall in love with long-distance running. She ran her first ultramarathon in 2008 and has been hooked ever since. Her favorite ultra are the timed events where she has fared quite well over the years: 110 miles in 24 hours at Hinson Lake in Rockingham, North Carolina, and 254 miles in 72 hours and 367 miles in six days, both at Across the Years in Glendale, Arizona. In her short tenure in the sport she has set several course records and hopes to set a few more in the years ahead.

Impressed? Me, too.

I trust this whetted your appetite for reading the book!

TAKING A MULLIGAN

SEPTEMBER 2015

When a golfer isn't satisfied with a shot they take another, commonly known as a mulligan—a chance to do it again for a better result. That is to say, *potentially* for a better result.

I played golf for more than 40 years, and I can honestly say I've taken my fair share of mulligans. As a runner for almost that same amount of time I've never had the luxury of a mulligan. What's done is done. But what if I could have done things differently... what might I consider changing that may have provided a better result?

- I've always had second thoughts about **starting a consecutive-days running streak** back in November of 1978. Running every day was SOP in my 20s, 30s, 40s, and even for most of my 50s, but now that I've hit the big six-oh, more and more of my early morning runs are becoming a challenge. In my defense, I never planned on my running evolving into a streak; it just happened. Promise.

- I might have sacrificed some of my mileage and **done a little more speed work**. When I was in my prime I was satisfied with running 5Ks between 17 and 18 minutes and 10Ks between 36 and 37 minutes. My peers admonished me on a regular basis for not doing enough speed work and were forever challenging me to break into the 16-minute and 35-minute ranges, respectively, for those two distances. But as I didn't have a particular fondness for running intervals, fartleks, or hills and was perfectly content with my race times, speed work and I—for all intents and purposes—were pretty much strangers. In spite of that I'm proud of the fact that I qualified for the Boston Marathon when a 2:50 or better was required for entry. If there's one thing that trumps speed work its youth, and at one time the latter was on my side.

- I may have **altered my plan of attack for the Badwater Ultramarathon** in 2003. Over the course of 135 extremely hot and extremely hilly miles I became overly reliant on the chair, using one to sit for a spell many more times than was physically necessary. The brief stints in the chair satisfied a psychological and emotional need, but in no way did it satisfy a physiological or biological one. The chair was basically a crutch, and I know in my heart I could have lowered my finishing time by several hours without it. It may have also helped to know Badwater was not only a very, very hot course, but also a very, very hilly course as well, that way I could have adequately prepared for the three mountain ranges I had to negotiate as I ran through Death Valley.

- I may have also **avoided running on trails**, a path I deemed necessary to get me to Squaw Valley for a race I had absolutely no business trying in the first place, the Western States Endurance Run. Twice, as a matter of fact. I'm fairly certain the assorted and sundry injuries I've been dealing with for most of the last decade are a direct result of the punishment I subjected my body to running 162 miles (I DNF'ed the first time in 2004 and finished dead last in 2006) up and down the Sierra Nevada for somewhere in the neighborhood of a composite 46 hours. Beyond that there were too many falls to count during my training on similar trails in preparation for my two starts at

Western States. These days you won't find me running on any trails because I've been placed on Double Secret Probation by the Running Police, the Coalition of Park Rangers, and the Environmental Protection Agency (something about me washing blood off after a fall on the trails in some stream at one time); long overdue if you ask me.

Other running mulligans that have crossed my mind (in no particular order):

- Running fewer miles in a pair of running shoes before removing them from active duty (this may have reduced the wear and tear on my body over the years).

- Volunteering more often earlier in my running career. (I did more than my fair share of racing and far, far less than my fair share of volunteering.)

- Competing in more races of my favorite event, the 24-hour run. (However, in my defense, during my prime 24-hour runs were few and far between.)

- Lived more, laughed often, and loved always. (Isn't this on everyone's list?)

Recently a good friend of mine, Gary Griffin, sent me a note as he was getting ready to run 100 miles—maybe a little bit more—for what he says will be the last time. I met Gary at the Callaway Gardens Marathon in 2002, and a little over a year later he was part of my crew at Badwater. We've been friends ever since, have run countless miles together, and have supported one another as fellow runners, fellow race directors, and brothers-in arm.

In his note Gary wrote that while he was mowing his lawn he asked himself it he was to do it all over again what would he do differently. Here's what he had to say:

My sincere heartfelt response and deep desire that it would have been so:
I would have met Scott Ludwig 20 years earlier.

You changed my life in so many ways, Scott. You took me from be-ing an average marathoner and fairly decent ultrarunner (who had formerly been a decent marathoner but had lost the speed that required) to showing me that I could go beyond 50 miles and live to tell about it. You let me witness your toughness and in a strange sort of way, some of that became part of me. You gave me confidence that I could be more than I thought that I could out there...so many things that you led me to that I would never have done without you.

So this begs the question: What if I had met Scott Ludwig in 1982 instead of 2002? Would I be crippled for life and living in a wheelchair? Maybe. Would I have done far more 100s and com-pleted the Grand Slam and been down there in the 17-hour range for 100 miles? Maybe.

But, I am just glad that our paths crossed the way that they did some 15 years ago now for what happened after that.

I replied:
Gee, Gary—that might be the most flattering thing I've ever had said to me. That means a lot, particularly since I've really tried to give back to the sport over the years and even more so because it came from you.

Don't be surprised if parts of it end up on my headstone one day.

If we had met in 1982 there's no telling what you and I would have accomplished in running—particularly if we lived in the same area and had the chance to run together a lot.

No telling...but I›m certain one of us (probably both) would be, as you said, in a wheelchair.

Gary's note made me think back to the original question I asked myself: What might I consider changing that may have provided a better result? And the answer became perfectly clear.

Not one single thing.

EPIC EXHAUSTION

OCTOBER 2015

Preface: After months of planning, the Senoia 60 Distance Festival—an event designed to test a runner's limits by seeing how far they can push themselves over the course of 60 hours—was less than 12 hours away. I had every volunteer's assignment meticulously outlined and every detail of the event accounted for. Everything was ready, and I was so confident in my choreography that I would be able to compete in my own event.

That's when it dawned on me: The only thing not ready was me. Not only was I exhausted from the last week of preparation for the event—buying the food and drinks, marking the course, touching base with all the volunteers, assigning bib numbers, etc.—I didn't have any time to rest or focus on my own personal plan of attack for running for a very long time.

....

The night before the Senoia 60 Distance Festival I was asked about my goals between the 6 a.m. Friday start and the 6 p.m. Sunday finish.

Never being the type to broadcast my goals prior to the start of a running event I opted to type them on a piece of paper, fold it in an envelope, and ask that it not be opened until after the Senoia 60 had come and gone. I figured worst case I had plenty of time to come up with some plausible reasons why I was a complete and utter failure and why running for 60 hours was stupid.

Even if running for 60 hours was my idea in the first place.

Then again, it's not like I've never done stupid things before. This certainly wasn't my first rodeo: Running for 60 hours was just the latest in a long litany of really stupid things I've tried over the years. Some turned out pretty well; others left a lot to be desired. But one thing's for sure: They've all left me with something to remember them by. Fantastic finishes, beautiful locales, and wonderful people, to name a few.

Then there are the numerous scars, occasional aches, and lingering pains, to name a few more. I couldn't help but wonder what running for 60 hours would add to my résumé. But I was more than ready to find out.

I wanted to see if I could literally run to the point of exhaustion.

Let's get this party started

Here are a few things you should do if you're planning to run in a 60-hour event:

1. Let someone else be the race director.

2. Get a good night's sleep the night before the race.

3. Be healthy.

4. Be young (optional).

Let's see how I did. As I mentioned previously, the race was my idea so it should be no surprise that I was the race director. I woke up at 1:11 a.m. race morning; I had the alarm set for 3:20. I was in the worst physical shape of my life (more on that later). The only people who consider me young either voted for JFK or think I *am* JFK. I guess that makes me oh-for-four.

What the hell was I thinking?

At least I had Kelly to keep me company for the next 60 hours.

Friday

I've known Kelly for over 20 years. Her sense of humor and devil-may-care attitude keeps me in stitches, always a good thing. When we run together her relentless pace also keeps me in stitches, just not the same kind and not always such a good thing.

We ran side by side Friday for almost 60 miles, laughing, reminiscing, and wondering if we were going to be functional by Sunday. Keep in mind Kelly is much younger than I am, is in much better health, is *not* the race director, and slept like a baby the night before. You can imagine what was going through my brain. Evil thoughts of imminent doom and embarrassing failure in an event I created to test my limits; limits that might be reached well before I thought they would. I wondered to myself why I couldn't settle for a more reasonable timed event, like 12 hours or maybe even 24. I guess I've always been an overachiever. Let's see if I can put my money where my mouth should never have been in the first place.

We started by running the 8.05-mile loop (there was also a 2.45-mile option) that we ran almost entirely using a flashlight because it was still dark outside. We noticed the odor of a dead skunk around the two-mile mark and hoped it would be gone the next time we passed through. It wasn't. On our third loop it was still there with one noticeable difference: The skunk raised its head, looked directly at us, and had a "kill me" expression on its face. Apparently the skunk had been struck by a car but didn't die. From that point on we opted for the shorter loop so we wouldn't have to see the skunk suffer because none of us had the stomach for putting the poor creature out of its misery. Throughout the day we told the other runners we chose the shorter loop "because the skunk moved."

Kelly called it quits for the day around midnight. I opted for one more 8.05-mile loop (the skunk somehow managed to crawl off the asphalt road) with Patrick, another runner who stayed with Kelly and me most of the day. When Patrick hallucinated (blueberry bushes in the middle of the asphalt road!), he decided he needed some sleep when we finished the loop. Just as I was thinking how I'd never hallucinated in my life I saw two runners in the bushes on the side of the road exchanging gear. When I did a double-take they were gone. I bet you can't guess who else decided they needed some sleep; 67 miles would have to suffice for the first day.

Saturday

After sleeping for two hours on the concrete floor of the pavilion, realizing it was too cold (50 degrees) to sleep outside, and moving to the comfort of my truck for another two hours, I woke up around 6 a.m. Saturday morning only to discover I had a blister on the ball of my left foot. Not having had a blister since a cherry tomato appeared between my toes while running through Death Valley over 12 years ago I wasn't sure what to do. I took one of the safety pins off my race number and pierced the blister, but no blood or water came oozing out; only air. I still couldn't walk on my left foot. Then I wrapped my foot in duct tape, something I hadn't done since shredding my left foot while running in the Sierra Nevada over nine years ago; that didn't seem to make a difference either. Then Ron, who had run with Kelly, Patrick, and me quite a few miles on Friday told me he once wore a beer koozie over his sore foot in a race, and he was able to make it to the finish line. Luckily he had one in his van for me to try (along with enough clothing for two dozen wardrobe changes, every medicinal supply you can find in a drug store, and enough gadgets to open his own Radio Shack—the man could *live* in his van if he had to).

You may laugh, but the koozie worked like a charm. Here's how it's done (clip and save):

- Remove shoe and sock.

- Wear the koozie on the end of your foot* as you would place a condom on the end of a banana.

- Put sock and shoe back on.

- Run.

After running primarily the longer loop on Friday, we opted for the shorter loop on Saturday—it reduced the time between rest breaks by 70%—and ran quite a few of them with Dan, who would go on to win the event with 157 miles.

---

* *If your foot is wider than the koozie, slit one or two areas of the koozie and then wrap everything in duct tape. Duct tape fixes everything. Everything except size-10 blisters filled with air, apparently.*

For the most part the day was a blur, but I do remember Ron saying he was "slapped in the face with exhaustion" at some point. Kelly, however, misinterpreted what he said and wondered where someone found an egg sausage to slap him with, and before you knew it all of us were laughing so hard our stomachs hurt more than they already did from running for well over a day and a half.

I guess what I'm trying to convey is this: We were all getting a bit punch-drunk from being on our feet for so long.

In other words, everything and everyone was flat out hilarious. It almost made me forget how much pain I was in.

Almost.

Sunday

Four hours of oft-interrupted sleep in the truck, and I was ready to finish the last day with both barrels blazing. The home stretch…the last hurrah…I wanted to do everything in my power to author an appropriate denouement to my running career.

Earlier I mentioned I was in the worst physical shape of my life. What I mean by that is my body as a composite—all the moving parts from top to bottom—have never been more discombobulated than they are right now. It would be easier to list the body parts that don't hurt or ache than those that do:

- What doesn't hurt: My hair, my earlobes, and the soft flabby skin on my elbows.

- What does hurt: Everything else.

At least my foot koozie was still doing its thing (when all was said and done I ran a total of 85 miles with the koozie on my foot—quick, someone call Guinness). Kelly ran a personal best of 120 miles, all of them with me (prior to that the most I had ever run with one person was 100 miles, so this was a personal best of sorts for me as well).

I mentioned writing my goals for the event prior to the start, and I'll get to them right after I tell you about another goal I set in my delirium yesterday as I was laughing about Ron getting slapped in the face with an egg sausage: I wanted to run more than 140.6 miles. Why? Because that's the total distance of an Ironman (2.4-mile swim, 112-mile bicycle ride, 26.2-mile run), and I thought it would be neat to design a T-shirt with this on the front:

- You covered 140.6 miles and for 112 of them you were sitting on your butt? How cute.

And this on the back:

- I ran 151.9 miles at the Senoia Distance Festival. On foot.

(Sorry if I offended any triathletes. I just found it funny at the time. Still do, actually.)

I finished the weekend with (as I just mentioned) 151.9 miles, a total that achieved one of my goals: To run farther than I ever have before.

Another goal I achieved was to get ultras out of my system once and for all. After several years of trying, I believe I've finally been successful. I've had more than my fair share of ibuprofen, Vaseline, salt tablets, and aid station fare for one lifetime.

Another was to run myself literally to the point of exhaustion. I'll admit my mind got there first, but my body wasn't far behind. As I write this report four days later I'm still in recovery mode (both mind and body) and looking forward to when everything returns to being functional.

Finally, I wanted to go out with a bang as a race director. Based on the post-race comments of those in attendance, I believe I was successful. The Senoia 60 was the perfect three-day running weekend, if I do say so myself. I wouldn't change a thing.

In all probability, the Senoia 60 will be the last race I ever direct, the last ultra I ever run, and will serve as the perfect denouement to my running career.

I'm 60 years old.

It was the 60th race I've directed.

60 hours is the ideal window of time to test one's limits.

At least for me it was. I'm exhausted.

The Senoia 60 became part of the Darkside Distance Festival in 2016.
I was the race director.

I also competed in the event and ran 119 miles.

Three months after my heart attack. (Details to follow)

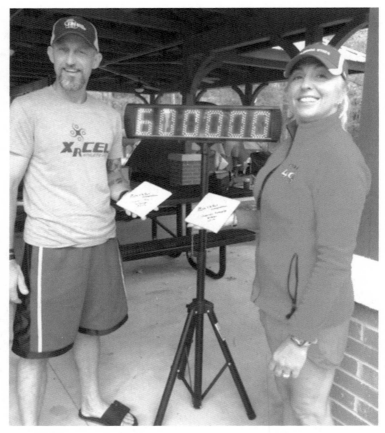

Dan Dunstan and Kelly Murzynsky, winners of the first Senoia 60

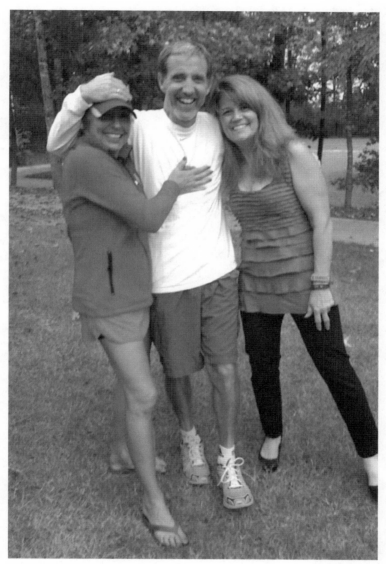

Kelly, Scott, and Valerie after spending 60 hours pounding the asphalt in Senoia, Georgia

NOVEMBER RAIN

NOVEMBER 2015

It started almost as a joke. "Paula's Big Butt 50K" we called it, the perfect way to celebrate the milestone birthday of Paula May, one of the original six members of the Darkside Running Club. It would also be the long overdue first ultramarathon—informal as it was—ever held in Peachtree City, Georgia, a running community interconnected by over 90 miles of runnable asphalt golf cart paths. The year was 2002, and the race was held on the second Sunday in November, my way of honoring the former Vulcan Marathon (Birmingham, Alabama), a race I loved running and really hated to see go by the wayside. *(While I'm on the subject: RIP Atlanta, Tybee Island, and Macon Marathons.)* Robert Youngren and Kelly Murzynsky were the men's and women's champions that inaugural year. It wasn't long before the Peachtree City 50K became an established and legitimate addition to the ultramarathon calendar in the southeast.

One short year later (2003), the Peachtree City 50K hosted the USATF Georgia Ultra Marathon Championship, and then transitioned to hosting the USATF National 50K Road Championship the following year. Mike Dudley won in 2004 and posted the fastest 50K time (3:05:34) of the year in the United States.

To celebrate our 10th anniversary, former Olympian Zola Budd Pieterse competed, setting a women's course record in the accompanying 25K (a distance added to the event in 2007).

The Peachtree City 50K (and 25K) has always offered a great value for a modest price. A beautiful course, enthusiastic volunteers, and a great group of runners has always been the norm. This, our 14th year, was no exception. Sophomore race director Heather Shoemaker (she took over for me in 2014) put on a wonderful event despite the most inclement weather in the history of the race: steady rain, 50-degree temperatures, and gusting wind. Yet the runners and the volunteers turned out in force and made, as the saying goes, lemonade out of lemons.

That's why it saddens me that this latest edition of the race will be its last. For reasons that have baffled me since the inception of the race, the Peachtree City 50K never established itself as a force to be reckoned with on the ultramarathoning running calendar. I do know part of that can be attributed to newly established marathons *(I'm looking at you, Columbus and Savannah!)*, muscling in on the second weekend in November, a sign of disrespect in this former race director's humble opinion. One positive impact of these infringing races has been our race has had its fair share of runners doing a double in recent years, running a marathon on Saturday and our 50K on Sunday. However, even in our most affluent years the total number of runners in both events rarely totaled much more than 100.

This year there were even less: 52 official finishers; 30 in the 50K, and 22 in the 25K. It never made sense to me why a runner would be willing to pay an entry fee upward of three times as much to run elsewhere; certainly the amenities couldn't be *that* much better than what we had to offer. And I sincerely doubt the personal attention the runners received from the volunteers at those aforementioned big ticket races could match what our event had to offer. I guess it boiled down to deciding between a small, intimate race offering the best (friendship, camaraderie, encouragement) of what running has to offer or a much larger event that all the cool kids are doing. To those who have opted for the latter these last dozen or so years, I have this to say to you: I'm sorry, but you simply missed out. And now you'll never know what you were missing.

I knew going into this year's event that Heather did not want to continue being race director. She grew a bit discouraged at how few runners signed up despite her diligent efforts to promote the event through various forums and outlets and doing whatever she could to take it to the next level. I know exactly how she felt; in fact, it's one of the main reasons I opted out of directing the race two years ago and was willing to let the race die a peaceful death. But as every runner knows, saying "never again" usually means "give it time, because probably there *will* be a next year."

But this year was different. I knew the exact moment when "never again" was never more definitive. It was 6 a.m. race morning. It was pitch black, pouring rain, and there was a damp coolness in the air that chilled me to the bone. I was dropping off the water coolers and tables for the mid-course aid station (affectionately known as Ice Station Zebra), standing in three inches of mud and using a handheld flashlight to see what I was doing. My work wasn't finished after setting up the tables; I then had to stand up the porta potty someone had knocked over during the night. Meanwhile the rain continued to fall and the wind continued to blow (neither of which would stop nor even slow down during the day). Throw in a bad case of the flu for good measure, and you have a pretty good idea of how I was feeling. It was at that exact moment I knew there was no hope of me believing that next year would be the year that the Peachtree City 50K would become a force to be reckoned with.

This year would be the last; there will be no next year.

But there is still this: The Darkside Running Club hosts several other events throughout the year offering the same intimacy, attention, and fun as the Peachtree City 50K. However, you'll no longer have the opportunity to compete on (arguably) the most recognizable 5.18-mile loop in the country in a race that began 13 years ago, almost as a joke.

While I am saddened the race will not go on, I'm proud of the accomplishments and perseverance of the runners (many who ran their first ultramarathon in Peachtree City), the contributions and dedication of the volunteers, and the impact the race had on the running community in its brief stay...not to mention the credibility it brought to Peachtree City as a viable ultrarunning community.

For the many of you who played a part in the history of the Peachtree City 50K:

Thank you.

Be sure to tell the others what they missed.

THE DEATH OF ME

NOVEMBER 2015

How many runners age 60 and over are running 10-plus miles a day?

As far as I'm concerned, the answer is one. That one would be me. There may be more, but I couldn't say for sure because I've never asked the question. And I've never asked the question because I don't really want to know the answer.

Knowing the answer could very well be the death of me, because regardless of how many miles they were running, I would want to run more.

Those who know me can attest that I'm a numbers guy. As fate would have it I chose a sport where performance is measured in numbers: How far...how fast...how many? I've had a lot of fun over the years tracking how far, fast, and many, but now that the first two are virtually untouchable and the latter is the only one that continues to (for lack of a better term) progress, numbers are beginning to lose their significance.

And that's a good thing, because otherwise numbers could very well be the death of me.

There was a time—somewhere in the neighborhood of 20 years ago—that I became obsessed with running as many miles as I possibly could. Monday through Friday I wasn't satisfied if I didn't run at least 11 miles in the morning before going to work. The weekends were for my long runs, typically back-to-back 20-milers on Saturday and Sunday with the exception of any Sunday that I knew of someone running more than 20 miles; on those Sundays, I would always make it a point to run farther.

It gets worse. On weekdays, I began running after work as well as before, usually another three to five miles (depending on how much I ate during the course of the day). If there were races on the weekend I would always opt for the longer distance (i.e., a marathon rather than a half), regardless of what kind of shape I was in or how rested I was ("wasn't" might be a better word). If I was going to end a day with 13.4 miles or a week with 108.6 miles, I made it my mission to run again and get those numbers up to 15 and 110, respectively. It's too painful to repeat what happened at the end of the year if, say, I wanted to reach 5,000 miles and I was a couple hundred miles short around Christmas.

That damn number fixation of mine could have been the death of me. I consider it a minor miracle that it wasn't.

If my friends and I went out for a 15-mile run, and we were met with heavy rain, thunder, and lightning shortly into our run and the rest of the group decided to cut the run short, I would finish out my 15 miles. If I had to be at work earlier than normal I didn't cut my run short; I merely set the alarm to ring earlier. (At that time "normal" was 2:30 a.m.) How does that saying go? I'll sleep when I'm dead?

The death of me, I say.

If nothing else, running for as long as I have has carved me out a relatively prominent spot on several running lists, lists that literally take someone a lifetime to make:

- Consecutive days running.

- Total lifetime mileage.

- Longest period between first and most recent ultra/50-miler.

There may be others, but these are the three with the most meaning, as they represent the fun and good fortune I've enjoyed over the many, many years of pounding the asphalt. Also keep in mind these lists have nothing to do with any particular skill or talent other than being able to stick with something for a really long time.

But lately running hasn't been all fun and good fortune. In fact, it wouldn't be wrong to say it's been exactly the opposite. I don't know which is worse—the physical ailments undoubtedly caused by overusing and abusing my body all those years or the chronic fatigue from too many miles and not enough sleep. What I do know is that if one day I intend to reach the top spot on the consecutive-days running streak I better set my sights on getting myself well in the very near future.

Besides, I want running to be fun again.

For that to happen, the first thing I need to do is stop running so much. Then I need to get more sleep. And for both of these to happen I need to drop my fixation with numbers, sooner rather than later.

Of course, if I reduce my mileage I may be in for a battle with another number: The number displayed on the bathroom scale.

So back to the original question: How many runners age 60 and over are running 10-plus miles a day?

As far as I'm concerned, the answer is none.

At least it will be once I get that number fixation out of my head.

RUNNING IS MY CHURCH

DECEMBER 2015

For many, many years the pastor of the church Cindy attended would ask me when I was going to start coming with her. I told him I had been attending church every Sunday morning—religiously, I might add—for more than a decade. Sure, I'd make it to church for an occasional Easter Sunrise or Christmas Eve service; other than that, my dance card on Sunday mornings was full. I had a standing date with the road.

Let me explain. I, along with my friends Al and Val, would meet early every Sunday morning at the local elementary school and run our requisite 20 miles—sometimes farther. We called it the Church of the Sunday Morning Twenty and attended come hell or high water (sometimes both).

But then the most amazing thing happened. Cindy found a new church she liked, asked me to try it on for size, and I did, and it fit. Not only that, the church held three services, the latter two giving me enough time to get in my Sunday morning long run.

It wasn't long before I was a regular. It wasn't long after that I was a volunteer at the information desk. The local newspaper printed a letter I wrote praising the charm, charisma, and virtues of the church.

Before long, 10 years had passed, and Cindy and I were established members of the congregation. Meanwhile the strangest transformation was taking place: I was seeing fewer and fewer members of the church Cindy and I had grown up with. I couldn't understand why anyone would leave such a charming and charismatic church.

And then one day it became abundantly clear. Let me explain.

The pastor was always very passionate about preaching that the number one reason people don't regularly attend church is because of their misperception that Christians are hypocrites.

From my tenure with the pastor's church I'm here to tell you that—at least in my situation—it wasn't a misperception. Not even close.

At first I thought it was just my imagination that the church staff was ignoring Cindy and me. Walking by us at our post at the information desk without looking in our direction, let alone saying good morning or simply sending a smile our way was how it started.

But it wasn't my imagination when the people in the church closest to Cindy and me turned out to be the biggest hypocrites of all. *Do unto others as you would have them do unto you* is how the saying goes. Well, if treating your friend with utter disdain and disrespect and using language better suited for a cameo in a remake of *Scarface* is how they want to be treated, this particular nail was hit squarely on its head. Because that's exactly how our "friend" treated us.

To be totally honest I can be quite an a** at times. In my defense, I'm only that way when the occasion calls for it. But under no circumstance would I ever stoop so low as to mock someone's mental competence, whether it's warranted or not. And I certainly wouldn't color those disparaging remarks with words better suited for the gutter.

Which is exactly what our friend—our hypocritical, degrading, and insulting "friend"—did.

Do unto others my a**.

I now understood why people were leaving the church. I don't need to tell you Cindy and I no longer belong to that church either, as charming and charismatic as it once appeared to us. Cindy has already started visiting other churches to find a new place to worship.

As for me, I don't need a pastor to tell me how to be a good person and do the right thing; my moral compass and conscience do a pretty good job in those areas.

I don't need to surround myself with hypocrites and backstabbers, not when I can spend time with true friends like Al and Val.

I don't need a large room with four walls and an altar to worship, not when I have endless miles of wide-open asphalt right in front of me.

For me running is—and always has been—my church. It's good for the soul.

Postscript: As I write this it's been nine months since I attended a Sunday morning service in my former church. Not one member of

*the church—staff or congregation—has taken the time to check in
on us to tell us we're missed or ask if we're OK.*

Sadly, I am not one bit surprised.

2016

SERIOUS AS A
HEART ATTACK

AN IMPERFECT 10

JANUARY 2016

Preface: The numbers presented in the following are necessary to illustrate the essence of this story. That is their sole purpose and intent. If for one second you think they are used for any other reason you would be dead wrong. My mileage pales in comparison to many, many, many runners I have come to know and admire. I always think back to when I first started running and read about a woman who ran 14,000 miles in a single year. From that perspective, anything I've ever accomplished is merely a drop in the ocean.

But should I ever run 14,000 miles in a single year, trust me, you'll hear about it.

But for now, I'm going with this.

Nadia Comaneci on the balance beam at the 1976 Summer Olympics.

Bo Derek in a swimsuit, running along the beach. In slow motion.

My score on every single 10-word spelling test I had in second grade.

All were perfect 10s.

I've always held a special fondness in my heart for nice round numbers. It's one of the side effects of an OCD personality, so I guess that special fondness is actually in my head rather than my heart.

That said, if there's a deadlier combination on this planet than a runner with OCD I can't imagine what it would be (other than human flesh trying to stop a speeding bullet or Eddie Murphy in any movie without *Beverly Hills Cop* in the title).

You want examples? Starting small and working my way up…

- It's becoming increasingly difficult for me to end a day on a non-round number. For example, if I were to run a 10K race (6.2 miles), I'll throw in some mileage with a .8 at the end to finish the day with a whole number. 6.2 miles + 2.8-mile warm-up or cool-down = 9.0 miles.

- There have been weeks when I realized I had a chance to reach a certain plateau (let's say 90 miles) and after Saturday's run I'd be at 77 miles with Sunday's run still left to finish off the week. Since Sunday has always been the day for my long run, it didn't make sense to run 13 miles and stop at 90. So I would run 23 miles on Sunday and finish at 100.

- Likewise, there have been months in which I followed a similar thought process—299 for the month with a whole week left would result in me running another 101 miles those final seven days. Many times I would wait until the last day of the month to check my mileage…again just to see if it was possible to finish the month on a nice round number. If the mileage needed was within reason (my definition of within reason and yours may not be the same), I considered it my duty to run what I deemed necessary (again, my definition of necessary).

- Don't think for one second that my annual mileage afforded me any luxuries. One year after my morning run on December 31, I was at an even 5,400 miles for the year. During the day I calculated my daily average to be 14.79 miles and discovered I needed to run another two miles to bring that average to an even 14.80. Don't think for one second I didn't do the math to figure out what I needed to raise it to an even 15.0. However, starting my second just before 5 p.m. didn't allow me enough time to run the requisite 75 miles so I just ran two miles and called it a year.

My first indication I might be able to kick my OCD to the curb occurred in 2006. I was running (for me) some really high mileage and was on the verge of averaging 13 miles per day for a span of 13 years. I surprised myself when I finished those 13 years averaging 12.99 miles a day. Believe it or not, I would have had to run an additional 47 or more miles on the very last day to raise my average a mere one-hundredth of a mile. But don't think for a second it was easy for me to dispel the notion of doing it.

My second indication of getting the OCD monkey off my back happened early last year when I noticed my monthly mileage was at 299 miles after my run on the last day of the month. I surprised myself when I chose not to run an additional mile to bring the total for the month to an even 300. *(As you may have suspected, I keep track of a lot of virtually meaningless numbers such as years with three, four, and five thousand miles; months with three, four, and five hundred miles; weeks with 80, 90, and 100 miles; and days with 10 miles or more. For several years I recorded the number of sit-ups I did each day—it always had to be a multiple of 50—and the number of beers I drank. OCD is a terrible thing. Or maybe it's a good thing. It's hard for me to tell, exactly.)* Believe it or not, it was easier deciding to *not* run that one mile than it was to brush off those 47-plus miles in 2006.

In no way, however, am I totally cured of my OCD. In 2015, I was very focused on the number of miles I wanted to run: 3,600. I simply wanted to average running 300 miles a month for the year just to show that someone 60 years old could. I was on pace for 3,600 miles throughout the year, but tried to get ahead of the game just a bit during the Christmas holidays as I knew Cindy and I would be spending the last two days of the year in the cabin of her brother and his in the mountains of North Carolina, not the easiest place to run. I did so well during the holidays I reached my goal several days before New Year's Eve. However, that posed another dilemma: Should I try to run 3,650 miles so I can say I averaged 10.0 miles per day as a 60-year-old? After my morning run on December 31, my log showed I was at 3,629 miles, or 9.94 miles a day. The thought of running another 21 miles (my morning run consisted of eight miles; eight very hilly, very challenging miles) was on my mind most of the day, up until the time the sun set, and I turned my attention to watching college football.

As I said, I'm not totally cured, but I'm certainly making progress. I felt pretty good (translation: I didn't dwell on it) about not finishing 2015 with 3,650 miles. As I do every year, I reported my annual and lifetime mileage to Steve DeBoer* who in turn posts this information on the runeveryday.com website. Steve noticed

---

* *Remember what I said earlier about my mileage paling in comparison to others?*
Steve has run more lifetime miles than me, and his consecutive-days running streak has me by a few years.
Also, I've always prided myself on not needing to run in tights unless the temperature dropped below 10 degrees Fahrenheit.
Steve uses the same criteria to determine when he needs to run in a shirt.

a discrepancy in my mileage from the prior year's tally, and after I thoroughly dissected my running long I discovered a mistake: I shorted myself eight miles in 2015. In other words, I would have only needed 13 more miles the afternoon of December 31 to reach 3,650 miles for the year.

On the plus side, my average miles per day elevated to 9.96 miles that, when rounded up, is an imperfect 10. However, the feeling in my stomach when I realized I was *this close* to a perfect 10.0 was all I needed to know about my OCD: It is still very much alive in me.

My remaining statistical goals at this time are to extend my consecutive-days running streak to 40 years and to reach 150,000 lifetime miles by my 64th birthday.

If I can reach both of those, anything else would be icing on the cake.

That is, as long as my OCD is gone by then.

MYTH BUSTER

JANUARY 2016

Cindy and I attended our annual Home Owners Association (HOA) meeting the other night. After the meeting, we met a couple who had recently moved into the neighborhood. The wife asked me if I was the person running in front of her house every morning. When I said, *"guilty as charged,"* she mentioned that she ran, sometimes as far as three miles. Then she asked me how much I ran.

At the same time Cindy and I both said the exact same two words: *Too much.*

The wife came back with this: *You can never run too much.*

Cindy and I had similar thoughts in our minds regarding her comment, a fact we found out later in the evening when we were able to talk alone. We both thought I was living proof that you can never run too much is nothing more than a myth.

....

Once upon a time there was a runner who woke up every day and couldn't wait to head out the front door for his morning run. In fact, he loved his morning run so much he didn't miss it for many, many years. He couldn't imagine what his day would be like if it didn't begin with a run. Fortunately, it was a moot point because he never missed a run, even if every couple of blue moons the thought of skipping a day crossed his mind. Heck, no one's perfect. But that thought never lasted for very long; only as long it took until he headed out the door for his next run.

Until one day the runner noticed he wasn't as excited as he used to be when his alarm went off precisely at 3 a.m.—as it had every weekday for as far back as he could remember. It became harder and harder to take that first step out the front door. Many days he took that first step only to adhere to an established timetable that allowed him to get his daily run in and still get to work on time. Sure, once he had a couple of miles under his belt he had that all-too-familiar feeling of being able to run forever. It wasn't long before he found it was taking more and more miles to achieve that same feeling; the joints just didn't loosen up like they used to.

And before he knew it, the feeling of being able to run forever was gone. He couldn't imagine what had changed. He examined the running logs he had meticulously maintained for over 30 years, searching for answers. It wasn't long before he noticed he had been making the exact same entries week after week for quite some time:

- Monday: 3:50 a.m., 8 miles

- Tuesday: 3:50 a.m., 8 miles

- Wednesday: 3:50 a.m., 8 miles

- Thursday: 3:50 a.m., 8 miles

- Friday: 3:50 a.m., 8 miles

- Saturday: 6:05 a.m., 13 miles

- Sunday: 6:05 a.m., 15 miles

- Weekly total: 68 miles

He couldn't help but notice the comparison to Jack Nicholson's "All work and no play makes Jack a dull boy" typed on page after page in *The Shining* as he was slowly but surely losing his mind. The only thing that varied from one week to the next was the weather conditions. He thought if his life were made into a movie it would be running's answer to *Groundhog Day.*

It was evident the runner was in a rut. Besides that, he was feeling more fatigued from running a mere 68 miles a week than he was several years ago when he was running well over 100.

Then it dawned on him: That time wasn't several years ago; it had been almost an entire generation. The runner was getting older, and the fatigue was simply his body's way of telling him to slow down. As he thought about it more and more, he couldn't help but think his body may have been trying to tell him that for years, but he just hadn't been interested in listening.

Now he was listening, but it wasn't as if he had any other choice. His body had now resorted to screaming. After all, talking never seemed to have any effect. The screams were telling the runner he wasn't running less, sleeping more, or doing one thing differently than he had for many, many years, and his body needed a break.

After giving the matter serious, serious thought, he decided he had to make a change. He had literally reached the point of exhaustion and knew that without a change he could quite possibly—and quite literally—run himself into the ground.

It was—without the slightest doubt whatsoever—now or never. It was time for him to slow down.

It was time for him to do something he had forgotten how to do: Rest.

....

The day after the HOW meeting, I placed a copy of my book, *Running Ultras to the Edge of Exhaustion,* on my new neighbors' front porch. The book chronicled the years I ran myself to the edge of exhaustion each and every day toward the completion of my personal Grand Slam of Ultras: The JFK 50, the Badwater Ultramarathon, the Western States Endurance Run, and the Comrades Marathon.

Inside the cover I wrote the following:

Proof that it's possible to run too much.

The neighbor sent me an email the following day thanking me for the book and referring to me as her crazy neighbor. It was also evident she had skimmed through the book because she added this:

You were right.

....

Running Out of Gas is a sequel to that book. It's the perfect depiction of how I feel at the end of my day. Not most days, but every day.

If I'm ever asked to appear in court to dispel the myth that it's impossible to run too much, I don't think I'd have much of a problem. All I would have to do is present Exhibit A.

Me.

Postscript: When I do appear in court to dispel the myth, I'm taking a copy of this book with me.

A PERSPECTIVE ON PERSPECTIVE

FEBRUARY 2016

I realize it's difficult for a runner to talk about running without dropping numbers. After all it's practically impossible to tell someone what you've accomplished in a pair of running shoes without them *(still talking about numbers here—not running shoes because some runners run barefoot, wear sandals, etc.)*.

It wouldn't make much sense to tell your neighbor you ran a race of considerable distance because that's about as vague as telling them you don't pass gas much. Rather, stating you ran 6.2 miles in less than 60 minutes and your pace was just less than 9 minutes per mile makes much more sense and is a lot easier for your neighbor to grasp. Plus, any neighbor who isn't tuned in to running is going to find your accomplishment impressive, mainly because you were able to do something they can't (and most likely because it's something they've never done and have no inclination to ever try) and have no earthly idea if your accomplishment is good, bad, or indifferent.

This is where I come in.

What if you had a neighbor who ran track or cross-country in college and was at one time capable of a 32-minute 10K? While this neighbor may not find your time impressive, any runner (or former runner) worth his or her salt will congratulate you nonetheless. Because that's what runners do: They support one another, even if they have to bite their collective tongues to do it.

What do I mean by "bite their collective tongues?" It's actually quite simple. If I've learned anything over the miles and the years I've been running it's this:

No matter what you've accomplished in your running career, there's someone else who has done it longer, farther, faster, and more often than you ever dreamed possible.

Here are a few examples to illustrate my point. Feel free to use them later to put your thoughts and impressions about running back into perspective. After all, that's been my intent from the start:

- Runner A tells a neighbor he drove his car to the garage to have some work done, ran the 17 miles back to his house, and would later run the 17 miles back to the garage when his truck was ready. Runner A's neighbor just so happens to be a friend of Ray Zahab, who ran 4,660 miles in 2006 across the Sahara Desert in 111 days (an average of 42 miles a day).

- Runner B tells a neighbor she ran four marathons in the past 12 months. Runner B's neighbor just so happens to be a friend of Dean Karnazes, who ran 50 marathons in 50 consecutive days in 50 states in 2006. Runner B's neighbor also knows Larry Macon, finisher of 239 marathons—all of them in the same year (2013).

- Runner C tells a neighbor he ran every single day for an entire six months. Runner C's neighbor just so happens to be a friend of Mark Covert, who recently ended a 45-year streak (that began in 1968) of running every day. Runner C's neighbor also knows Jon Sutherland, who assumed the longest active running streak in the country less than a year after Mark Covert ended his in 2013.

- Runner D tells a neighbor she managed to complete a 100-mile run, the hardest thing she's ever done. Runner D's neighbor just so happens to be a friend of Ed Ettinghausen, who ran 40 races of 100 miles or longer, all in the same year (2014). Runner D's neighbor also knows Mike Morton, who ran 100 miles at a pace quicker than eight minutes per mile, not to mention covering just over 172 miles in a 24-hour event on another occasion.

- Runner E tells a neighbor he qualified for the 100-mile Western States Endurance Run. Runner E's neighbor just so happens to be a friend of both Tim Twietmeyer (25 sub-24-hour finishes at Western States including five overall wins) and Ann Trason (14 wins at Western States).

Obviously in all five of these examples there exists an entire spectrum of performances between the numbers the runners dropped and the accomplishments of the various friends and acquaintances of their respective neighbors. As I said before, when you are talking about running you always need to keep things in perspective because there will always be someone who has done it longer, farther, faster, and more often than you.

Unless someone specifically asks you for your numbers…time, distance, pace…it doesn't matter; it's wise to keep them to yourself. Don't expose yourself to the risk of being one-upped.

It's a game where no one wins.

Just remember: When it comes to running the only one you must impress—the only one you *need* to impress—is you.

CURTAIN CALL

FEBRUARY 2016

My first marathon was in Gainesville. Now I can say the same thing about my last. I wouldn't want it any other way.

So much has happened since that first time back in 1979. The Florida Gator football team became a force to be reckoned with. Even the Florida Gator basketball team has made its mark on the national landscape of collegiate sports. Enrollment at the University of Florida has more than doubled. Way more, in fact; perhaps the allure of National Championships and year-round sunshine deserves some credit. And—sadly, the first I referenced earlier—the Florida Relays Marathon—no longer exists.

I was a 24-year-old graduate student who had never run farther than 13 miles. I knew more than doubling that mileage at one time would be a challenge, but I had no idea how much of one. I finished my first marathon that day with barely six months of running under my belt, and now one month shy of 37 years later I can say I finished my last. Sadly 1979 would also be remembered as the last edition of the Florida Relays Marathon.

But I didn't run my last marathon alone.

Flashback to one year earlier. My son Josh and I were on the starting line of the 10th annual Five Points of Life Marathon in Gainesville, Florida. He asked me to not only run it with him but also to pace him to a sub-four-hour finish. Although cautioning him he was being a bit optimistic with his time goal, I reluctantly kept him on pace to break four hours. For 18 miles, that is, because I was no match for what came next.

Josh came down with a bad case of the cramps from hell. Josh slowed down, walked, and finally hobbled the next four miles before finally taking a swan dive in the shade of the medical tent at the 22-mile mark. One of the volunteers—a retired doctor, incidentally—tended to Josh immediately, providing fluids and ice and making sure he was comfortable. He also gave him a litany of advice, most notably that his first marathon will have to wait.

Josh's eyes lit up. "I have to finish."

The good doctor looked at me and asked, "What do you think, dad?"

Josh knows me well enough to know that if I told him I thought it best he stop that I would be lying through my teeth. I'm just not very good at practicing what I preach when it comes to saying no or moderation to all things running. "I'm not the man for that," I said.

To my credit, though, I did add: "But he is probably right. You're in an awful lot of pain, and there's always another marathon."

Josh, to his credit and as testimony he has a lot more common sense than his dad, decided to take the good doctor's advice and call it quits after 22 miles and almost three-and-a-half hours under a warm Florida sun. As there was no sag wagon to transport Josh to the finish, it was up to me to finish out the last 4.2 miles of the race, get in the car, and drive back to the medical tent to pick him up.

A little over an hour later Josh and I met up with Cindy (who also saw me finish *my* first marathon in 1979) near the finish line for some post-race pizza and fluids when Josh, who knew prior to the start of the race that my intention was for it to be my final marathon, looked at me and said: "It looks like you have one more marathon left to run."

Being the most susceptible person in the world to the power of suggestion I immediately knew Josh spoke the truth. That explains why I kept my mileage up—I would run more than 3,700 miles over the next 12 months—when all I really wanted to do was reduce my mileage to something more appropriate for a man approaching middle age (assuming I'll live to be 120, that is).

Twelve months later and there we were: On the starting line for the 11th annual Five Points of Life Marathon in Gainesville on a warm February morning. Josh hadn't put in the mileage like I had, but then again, his legs were half as old as mine and had a lot less wear and tear on them. I guess what I'm trying to say is we were pretty much on equal ground, and this year our one and only goal was to finish like a seat on an airplane during landing: in the upright position.

Running with our good friend Ferit Toska, a three-hour marathoner, I have to admit it turned out to be one of the most pleasant and enjoyable 26.2-mile runs (if that's even possible) I've had in a very, very long time. We took occasional breaks at the aid stations, took in all the sights, and even managed to synchronize all of our pit stops. No one ever fell behind or pulled ahead. It went by so fast it was almost painless, although the day after would make it clear to Josh and I that it was anything but. Ferit is another story, but then again, he's in his marathoning prime at the moment so he doesn't really count.

The highlight of the marathon was stopping at the medical tent at 22 miles and asking that very same doctor if he remembered me from last year. "Your son!" he said. "He's right behind you," I replied. The three of us posed for a photograph before the good doctor wished Josh well and told him he was glad he returned to give the marathon another chance. As we resumed our pace I thanked him for keeping Josh's spirits up and looking out for him twelve months earlier.

We ran (and to be honest, walked once or twice) almost four miles where we met up with my grandson (and Josh's nephew) Krischan who would join us for the last third of a mile to the finish line. While the original plan was for Krischan, Josh, and me—representing three generations of our family—to cross the finish line simultaneously, my grandson sped up when he saw the finish line and had his first official "marathon finisher" photo taken. Josh, Ferit, and I crossed the finish line together that made for a memorable photo that I intend to have framed—along with his finisher's medal, of course—for him. I might do the same for me. If I do I'll set it next to the trophy I won—the first trophy I ever won in a marathon—at the 1994 Vulcan Marathon. Josh, only nine years old at the time, rode his bicycle alongside me that cold November Sunday in Birmingham, Alabama, the entire 26.2 miles, so the Five Points of Life Marathon wasn't the first time the two of us crossed a marathon finish line together.

My close friends had asked me prior to the marathon to post a photo on social media once we finished. I obliged with a photo of Josh, Krischan, and me—all in our Darkside Running Club shirts and sharing two medals between the three of us—and a caption stating it was Josh's first marathon…and my last.

If there's one thing I've learned in running it's to listen to the advice of the grizzled veteran runners, a group I now consider myself a part of. Gary Griffin, a long-time friend, fits that bill as well. He wrote beneath my caption:

"If this is IT, what a way to go out, huh?"

I couldn't agree more.

Postscript: One day, Krischan may decide to run a marathon. I will more than likely be in my 70s by then. Right now, I've run a marathon in five different decades (my 20s, 30s, 40s, 50s, and 60s), an accomplishment shared by my good friend (and another grizzled veteran of running) Al Barker. It's tempting thinking about one-upping him by running a marathon when I'm 70. However, he, too, has offered me countless advice about running and aging through the years, and this one sticks out in my mind right about now:

It's time to rest on your laurels.

Once again, I couldn't agree more.

My first was in Gainesville. Now I can say that about Josh's first as well as my last.

I wouldn't want it any other way.

Fin.

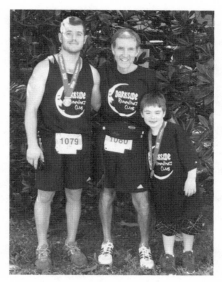

Josh, Scott, and Krischan after crossing the finish line of Josh's first marathon in Gainesville, Florida

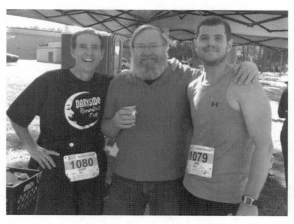

Scott and Josh "reminiscing" with the good doctor one year later

RUNNING UNDER THE INFLUENCE

APRIL 2016

I was running with three other members of my Darkside Running Club—Valerie, Keith, and Kristen—at our Running Dead Ultra (50K, 50-mile, and 100-mile options) when Keith looked at Valerie and me and asked how long the two of us had been running together. Valerie said she and I started running together in the summer of 1993 to prepare Valerie to run the Atlanta Marathon (and earn a Boston Marathon qualifying time) on Thanksgiving Day. We've been running together ever since.

Keith said, "*boy, I bet you have some stories.*" I politely mentioned some of them have been chronicled in my books. Valerie added that there were plenty more…that I *didn't* write about. Like the Labor Day 10K in Macon back in the mid-1990s…

Flashback

Valerie, Al (another long-time running partner), and I made the 90-minute pilgrimage to Macon where we spent the night to rest up for one of our favorite annual events as it offered many amenities other races didn't. At the top of the list: a fast course, a reasonable entry fee, and the opportunity to get hammered before 10 a.m.

Once upon a time the Macon Labor Day races (both 5K and 10K distances are offered) essentially provided all the beer you could drink. If you were wearing your race number in the park at the finish, you could get as many unopened bottles of beer as you wanted. In 1994, among Valerie, Al, and me, that number turned out to be 23, all by 10 a.m. It would have been more but the vendor ran out of beer. The noise generated by 23 empty glass bottles as we carried them in a plastic trash bag to the garbage can caught everyone's attention (as we were told much, much later) and made an impression that would change the course of history at the Macon Labor Day Road Race (it wasn't long before beer was no longer offered after the race). We failed to anticipate what the combination of running as fast as we could for 6.2 miles in the heat and humidity of Macon, Georgia, and drinking a cumulative 288 ounces of beer were doing to us; that wouldn't come until we stood up to run back to the start where we had parked our cars— six-point-two miles away—four hours earlier.

It took seemingly forever to get back to our cars, and at least one of us got us lost so many times the 6.2-mile return trip ended up being almost 10 miles. (Let me add the course looks a lot different running it in reverse, especially after one's fair share of 23 beers.) One of us had to use a restroom *really bad* and had to settle for the side of a building—in full view of a random stranger or two—because there wasn't a restroom or porta-potty in site the entire run back to the car (again I can't remember whom, but I will tell you it was the first time he or she went number 1 standing up). Finally, one of us extended their hotel stay in Macon a second night so the effects of their third of the alcohol would wear off. The other two somehow if not downright miraculously made the 90-minute drive back home. I won't say who the two were, but I will tell you Al had a wonderful three-hour nap.

Return to the Present

Valerie said to Keith, Kristen, and me that she and I should write a book. We discussed possible titles; the really good ones won't be listed here so that this story's PG rating can remain intact.

A short while later Valerie had to leave as she had to show some houses to a client of hers (Valerie is a realtor). As Valerie drove by the three of us as we continued running she called me over and said, "*running under the influence*," a reference to that day in Macon almost a generation ago. I instantly loved it as a title and told her I was using it, and that she'll be seeing it in writing very soon.

As Valerie drove away I mentioned the phrase to Keith and Kristen. They loved it as well, albeit with a slightly different interpretation. Keith said he wouldn't be here today running 50 miles if it weren't for me. Kristen said the same. For whatever reason that felt really good to hear; something I had said or done had influenced them into running 50 miles on this beautiful spring day.

I spent a good bit of the day thinking about what they said. Hundreds of feelings and emotions ran through my mind; so many that it was virtually impossible to isolate one that stood out the most. Flattered? Humbled? I simply couldn't put my finger on the right word.

Reflections

Later that day I thought about what Keith and Kristen had said. It made me think of other possible influences I've made over the past 38 years in the running world:

- Runners who became members of the club Al and I founded in 2002, the Darkside Running Club

- Runners I've paced in marathons to earn a qualifier for the Boston Marathon

- Runners who finished their first marathon/ultramarathon in a Darkside event

- Runners who have been successful following tips they've gathered from me—whether it's something I've said, something I've written, or something they've seen me do*

- Runners who have started a running streak (I would never recommend this, incidentally. I've got almost 38 years of reasons why.)

- Runners who have been motivated by reading my books about running, my blogs about running, or my columns in running magazines

- Runners who said they were inspired after hearing me speak at a running function

- Runners who have volunteered after seeing how hard the volunteers at Darkside events work to make sure every runner has a good experience

- Taking it a step further, runners who have become race directors after being inspired at a Darkside event

- My written words being used by others ("Running is a privilege," "if you say you're going to do it, you've got to do it,"

---

* *I never offer running advice unless I'm specifically asked;*
   what works for me may not work for someone else.

"run a 20-miler each week so you're in marathon shape year-round," and "premature acceleration," which means starting out much too fast in a race and slowing way down toward the finish)

- Runners who pass on my running adventures and experiences to others

- And best of all, nonrunners who became runners because they—in some way, shape, or form—were influenced by my running

As the dust settled later that day I got a phone call from my son Josh. Two short months ago he ran his first marathon, something he promised me he would do when he was 17 years old (he's 30 now). I was with him every step of those 26.2 miles. It just so happened that today he ran his first ultramarathon, a 50K in a location not too far away from where I held today's Darkside event. It made me think of something Josh said to Al when he was only seven years old: *"When I grow up I want to be just like my dad."* In two short months Josh had become a marathoner as well as an ultramarathoner, just like his dad.

After speaking with Josh, I opened the local newspaper and saw that the Huddleston Hustle, a small 5K in Peachtree City, was run that morning. The Huddleston Hustle was first held in 2002 and back then was known as the Run for Alex. I should know— I helped establish it with my next-door neighbor Stephanie. The race was a tribute to the memory of her son Alex who lost his battle with leukemia while still a student at Huddleston Elementary School. The proceeds of the race went to books for Alex's corner, a part of the school library where Alex liked to read. It was comforting to know the race was still going strong in its 15th year, partially because I was a part of it in the early years but even more so because of the reason it was created in the first place.

Two days later Ed Ettinghausen, who ran the 100-mile version of the Running Dead Ultra, spoke to the employees at my distribution center. He spoke about his life, his keys to success, and a word or two about his running. (Ed currently has the world record for most races of 100 miles or more completed in a calendar year—40. He is also an accomplished motivational speaker. And those are just the tips of an enormous iceberg.) Before his presentation I introduced him to Antonio, a man I've worked with for as long as I can remember. Antonio has volunteered at more than his fair share of Darkside events over the years. I mentioned to Ed that Antonio had just started running. Antonio told him about the running shoes he bought recently—his very first pair, by the way—with the giddiness of a first-time father talking about his newborn child.

Coincidentally, at the time Ed was speaking to my employees the last runner I paced to their first Boston Marathon qualifier, Ami Lewis Roach was competing in her fourth Boston Marathon. I remember running 26.2 miles with Ami in Birmingham back in 2011 in my pacing finale and how excited *both* of us were when she crossed the finish line with a qualifying time.

When I got home that evening Antonio—as he's been doing the last two weeks ever since he started running—sent me a text message with the distance, time, and pace of his latest run: 2.20 miles, 21 minutes and 16 seconds, and a pace of 9:21 per mile. I replied, "you're making me look bad." He replied, "I'm going to make you proud one day."

I texted him back, "You already have."

And then it hit me. That was the word I was looking for earlier. Proud.

I'm proud of what I've been able to contribute to the sport of running.

That nasty little incident in Macon aside, of course.

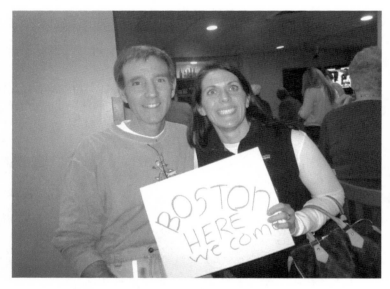

Scott and Amy, the last person Scott paced (in Birmingham, Alabama) to a Boston Marathon qualifier

THE RUNNING WIDOW

MAY 2016

"You're getting fat. You need to start running."

—Cindy Ludwig, summer of 1978

So what if I put on a couple of pounds? The truth of the matter is it wasn't even my fault.

We were newlyweds living in married housing at the University of Florida. We were both attending graduate school, and I had a part-time job at the local Burger King where one of the perks was getting to eat for free on the days I worked. In other words, a Whopper, large fries, and a vanilla shake were at my beck and call four (sometimes five) times a week. And since we were on a budget at the time, free meals were a really big deal.

Meanwhile I was monitoring my weight religiously because I had a slight suspicion those four (sometimes five) calorie-laden meals every seven days might add up over time. The needle on the scale didn't seem to be moving too far to the right, and the fact I was buying larger pants every six weeks or so never sunk in. Then one day, Cindy asked me if I realized the scale was using kilograms as its unit of measure (I didn't) and to make a really long and embarrassing story short the, weight I thought I was (168 pounds) was actually 88 kilometers...or 194 POUNDS!

Again, let me reiterate that it wasn't entirely my fault. Blame Burger King and a possible nationwide conversion to that inane metric system we were threatened with back when I was in school.

So I took Cindy's advice and started running. Six months later I was down to 150 pounds and buying pants with the same waist-line I wore when I was 13. Now almost 40 years later my weight remains around 150 pounds, and I'm still running. So if you look at it from that perspective, the fact that I run isn't necessarily my fault either; more so Cindy's. As for running every day since 1978—well, that's entirely my fault because OCD is a b*tch and never wants to take the blame for *anything*. Yep, that one's on me.

To be sure, running every day has proven to be difficult at times. There have been countless reasons for missing a run over the years, yet I've laced up my running shoes every single day, some days more than once. But I didn't do it alone.

I couldn't possibly have done it without Cindy. If there is such a thing as a running widow, it would have to be her. For your con-sideration:

- I wake up at 3 a.m. during the week to run and leave for work before Cindy wakes up, then I normally pass out by 9 p.m., if not earlier. That doesn't give us much time to be together since she doesn't get home until 8. In other words, we spend about four hours during the week with one another. I would have to be dead or gone for it to be much less. Yet she never complains about the four or five hours every night during the week she spends alone.

- Over the years I've been away at least a portion of more than 800 weekends to run a race. In the earlier days that would con-stitute several hours on a Saturday morning for a local 5K or 10K; in the later days, an entire weekend to run nothing less than a marathon, most of them in another city, state, or in some cases country. Yet Cindy never complains about spending the day (and in some cases more than one) alone.

- As I always seem to be in a constant state of fatigue and am prone to falling asleep whenever my head rests against anything (a pillow, the back of a couch, the floor), Cindy has never complained about it—even the times when I've done it at the home of one of our friends or that one time in a meeting with our oldest son's second grade teacher while sitting in a chair.

Aside from all the time she's spent (for lack of a better word) alone, she's also:

- Run a little bit herself, including 30 half marathons and one particular 10K while pregnant with our first son.*

- Volunteered to help with many of the races I've directed in way too many capacities to list here.

- Made the trip to Honolulu to see me finish my 200th marathon, which was also going to be my last.**

- Patiently yet reluctantly allowed me to run 60 miles for my 60th birthday; my last big thing, as well as the last big thing after that: Running for 60 hours after I turned 60 years old.

---

* *She didn't find out she was pregnant until a couple of days after the race, so didn't know she could have won the prize for the fastest time by a pregnant lady presented by Rod Dixon, the only world-class runner Cindy has ever had any interest in meeting.*

** *There have been a few more since then.*

Out of everything Cindy has done to demonstrate her support for my running over the years, the thing that stands out most is that she understands what I'm doing and what I go through every time I head out for a run. I know this to be true because as I was preparing to run 135 miles across Death Valley in the summer of 2003, someone asked Cindy if she was going to be going along with me as part of my support team. Her reply said everything I needed to know that she truly does understand:

"I know Scott will be in pain at times, and I'd have a hard time containing my emotions. I wouldn't want him to see that because that would be bad for him."

These days I'm running fewer miles and fewer races and spending a lot more time on things you would expect a sexagenarian *(hey now)* to do. Working on household projects, spending time with the grandchild, and sitting on the front porch watching the world go by are at the top of my list at the moment. As for my running, all that remains is a certain mileage goal that will not be mentioned here and a goal of one day owning the longest consecutive-days running streak in the world. To make those happen all I'll need are two things: (a) some semblance of health and (b) a pulse.

Other than that, I'm pretty much taking it easy and ready to do all the things Cindy and I have wanted to do since we started dating during our senior year in high school. No longer will she be the running widow.

Just as soon as I take care of a few remaining loose ends.

MAKING MEMORIES IN MORELAND

MAY 2016

If there is one thing I've learned about the Darkside 8-Hour Run since its inception in 2003 it is this: There will be one indelible moment that everyone will remember. Whether it's the torrential lightning and thunderstorm that resulted in a one-hour interruption and a subsequent three inches of water on the Riley Field track, the 40-degree weather and accompanying rain, wind, and hail (*in May, no less*) the first time the event was held at Bear Creek Farm, or the event-record performances of Eileen Torres (54.06 miles) and Ferit Toska (56.1 miles) in 2014, the event always leaves something behind that people will be talking about in the years ahead.

This year the event was held at beautiful Bear Creek Farm in Moreland, Georgia, for the fourth consecutive year...and this year, the event more than lived up to its reputation. I'll get to that later, but first I want to share what turned out to be one of the most enjoyable running experiences of my life.

I had the privilege to run at least one loop (1.02 miles) with almost everyone in the event at one time or another, some of them I've known seemingly forever and others I was meeting for the very first time. To be honest it was really hard to tell because in running everyone is family; there are no strangers.

In no particular order (*I'd be hard pressed to list them any other way*) I ran with:

- Debbi, a former Darkside 8-Hour champion whom I hadn't seen in a couple of years. She was running as strong as ever, and we talked about the good old days (*before our bodies started to betray us*) and how good one another looked (*she was lying; I wasn't*).

- Ron, who always tells me how much he doesn't like to read but enjoys my articles—the short ones, anyway. I told him when I write I always can tell when I'm past the point of keeping his interest and that I was writing a book of short stories (*working title "Short Attention Span Theater"*) and that when it's published it will be dedicated to him. (*True story.* If you're looking for fiction, read Stephen King. That or my first work of fiction, *Best Foot Forward*.)

- Beth #1, another former 8-Hour champion who will be crewing for another runner in Death Valley in two months at the 135-mile Badwater Ultramarathon and depending on how things go, may consider running it herself next year. If she does she asked if I would be on her crew (*naturally I agreed because I rarely have the presence of mind or requisite common sense to say no*).

- Beth #2, whom I hadn't seen since she became a mother of two but seemed to have way too much spring in her step to be a mother of two. Every time she passed by me (*more times than I care to remember*) the thought "motherhood suits her" crossed my mind. She nodded and said, "gentle dude" every time in return to my thought bubble, which would have been the coolest phrase of the day if it hadn't been for my grandson (*to be continued...*).

- Heather and Patrick, who will be getting married next month (*they met for the first time at a Darkside event a couple years ago*). Incidentally, their ceremony will be at 6:30 on a Saturday morning and will be followed by an 8-hour race of their own.

- Adamy, who will be helping me with the Darkside Distance Festival this October. I found out she—like me—thinks clearer when she runs and came up with several good ideas for the event for me to consider.

- Ferit, the event record-holder with whom on this day I managed to run side by side…for one loop, anyway. A little while later I had almost as much trouble keeping up with Ferit's son Derin for a loop, who apparently has a good bit of his dad's genes (*thank goodness I have more endurance than most four-year-olds).*

- Krischan, my seven-year-old grandson who took up where he left off last year when he called everyone he passed out on the course "slow pokers." This year he not only called them slow pokers; he included "lazy boners" in his repertoire (*a phrase I absolutely loved—even more than "gentle dude"*).

At the end of the day, after eight hours of running the paved and rolling 1.02-mile loop of asphalt two former champions showed their mettle and finished with the most mileage: Ferit led all the men with 49.98 miles (*sorry, Ferit, 49 loops x 1.02 miles = 49.98 and we do not round up!*), and Beth #1 was the top woman with 43.86 miles. By the way, both of them were mentioned in my 2013 book *Distance Memories* as having incredibly bright futures in running. Color me clairvoyant.

As for me, I spent most of those eight hours running, filling water coolers, updating the leader board every hour, and simply enjoying the camaraderie only runners can share. I didn't have a particular goal in mind until Ferit reminded me that my next marathon or ultra would bring my lifetime total of those two distances to 262, a fitting number since a marathon is 26.2 miles. Ferit had suggested to me a couple months ago that I should run 262 miles to celebrate the occasion; I figured running 31 loops to constitute an ultra of 50 kilometers would get that thought out of his (*and my*) head. Additionally, someone told me a while ago that I was on a list of runners with the greatest amount of elapsed time between their first and most recent ultra. My first was the Stone Mountain 50-Mile Run on February 6, 1982, so after running 50K today my elapsed time between my first and most recent ultra would extend to 34 years, 3 months, and 8 days. (*Note: I have no idea where I stand on the aforementioned list but I do know it's in the top 100. Hell, it might be in the top 10 but don't ask me; I've never seen the list.*) I still remember the first official advice I received as an ultrarunner from Vaughn Crawley as I was running one of the severe uphills of my second (of 10) five-mile loop around the base of Stone Mountain: "*In ultras it's advisable to walk the uphills.*" I've never forgotten it.

Getting back to that one indelible moment...

I had the pleasure of running about a dozen laps with Antonio, a man whom I've known for over 20 years. He started running less than two months ago, a fact I know because he texted me every night with the mileage, the time, and the route he ran accompanied by an occasional question or two about the sport. At my suggestion, he started out by running two miles a day, quickly upping the ante to four. He developed a growing fascination with running shoes, asking me virtually every day at work about a particular brand or style to get my opinion. A couple weeks ago he ran his longest run ever: 6 miles. I encouraged him to run at Bear Creek just to get a feel for running with others and to enjoy the camaraderie. He took my suggestion and wasn't disappointed; neither was I.

Before heading to the starting line, he told me he hoped to run 10 miles so he could make me proud. I ran several loops with him and passed along the advice I first heard in 1982 at the base of the only uphill on the loop. He thanked me later and said how the short breather he got walking the uphill every loop reenergized him. After he finished his first 10 miles he walked another four with his wife Miriam. After that he started running again because now he had his sights set on bigger game: finishing a marathon. A few hours later he accomplished just that: 26 loops and 26.52 miles, qualifying him as one of the few people who technically ran an ultra before running a marathon. He had a smile on his face when he finished; the same one he started with over six hours earlier.

Antonio had quadrupled his longest run and gone from 2 to 26 miles in less than two months. I mention them both in a single sentence because I can't discern which is more impressive. Either way I was impressed...*very* impressed, and trust me when I tell you I don't say that very often.

Later that night Antonio sent me a text: *'Just wanted to tell you THANKS for everything. I've never been treated so good today by everyone!!!"*

The perfect ending to a perfect day: Antonio had discovered the camaraderie of running and the joy of fulfilling a dream.

As for me, number 262 is in the books. If it's the last marathon or ultra distance I ever run, I can't think of a better or more appropriate ending.

I can live with that.

LIFE SENTENCE

MAY 2016

For years people have asked me why I'm not fond of running on trails and why I have no interest in trying an Ironman. Thinking back, I believe the answers to both can be found in something that happened over half a century ago.

You would think a person who has played more than 2,000 rounds of golf in his life would love the great outdoors.

You would think a person who spent many a summer on the shore of the ocean or by the side of a pool would love the great outdoors.

You would think a person who has run well over 140,000 miles beneath sun and moon would love the great outdoors.

If you would think all those things you would be right. However, if you were to think that same person would love to spend ONE SINGLE NIGHT in the great outdoors you would be wrong. I'm convinced sleeping with a roof over your head is why God made beds; sleeping bags are the work of the devil.

I discovered how much I hated spending the night in the great outdoors when I was—of all things—a Cub Scout in Quonset Point, Rhode Island. Our Cub Scout pack went on a camping trip in the dead of winter to some remote god-forsaken mountain. Here's what I remember: snipe hunts, Vienna sausages, latrines, and sleeping in a lean-to that didn't protect me from the violent snowstorm we encountered during the night. Here's what else I remember: There was also no way to take care of the little things I'd grown accustomed to. Personal hygiene, for example. It was in all probability the most horrific weekend of my life. One last thing I never forgot: I swore I would never do it again.

Ironically a few years later I was the Senior Patrol Leader of my Boy Scout Troop in Honolulu, Hawaii. Don't be misled: I didn't earn the position; rather I "aged" my way into it. I had no business being a Boy Scout, let alone the leader of a whole troop of them. Yet somehow I worked my way through the ranks: Tenderfoot, Second-Class, First-Class, Star and Life, which is only one rank below the highest rank of all, Eagle Scout. I was even (miraculously) inducted into the Order of the Arrow, a society honoring scouts who best exemplified the Scout Oath and Law.

As for never reaching the rank of Eagle Scout…

To become an Eagle Scout back then you had to earn 21 merit badges: 14 required and 7 elective. I was only one required merit badge short of cashing in; lifesaving was the only thing holding me back from flying with the Eagles. Although never a particularly good swimmer, I somehow swam well enough to earn the swimming merit badge. Once I even swam a whole mile, although I did have to hang onto the side of the pool after every 25-yard lap—which was a lot better than the other option (drowning).

However, lifesaving was another story. One of the requirements was to jump in a pool fully clothed, remove your shirt and blue jeans, and swim to the side. This one I completed. I was also required to swim 50 yards manually towing a life-sized dummy as if I were saving it from drowning. This one I could never complete.

To visualize how well that went imagine a rather large leaf float-ing in a lake; then mentally throw a brick on top of it. I was the leaf.

I never got past that final hurdle to Eagle Scout-dom. A dummy stood in my way. Today the Boy Scouts of America still require the Lifesaving merit badge for the rank of Eagle Scout...OR the Emergency Preparedness merit badge. For the latter, rather than actually *swimming*, all you have to do is show how you could safely save a person from drowning, using non-swimming res-cues.

I feel pretty certain I can flag down a lifeguard or scream really, really loudly for help.

But that's all water under the bridge now. I'll have to be content being a Life for life.

THE THIRD RULE

JUNE 2016

Running, like most any sport, is governed by numbers. Miles, kilometers, meters…hours, minutes, seconds…heart rates, BMI, stride length…how far or how short…how fast or how slow… whatever it is, numbers rule the sport of running.

And like any sport, running has its fair share of numerical rules and axioms. For example:

- When you begin running, limit your weekly mileage increases to no more than 10% a week. For example, if you start out running 20 miles a week, you should target no more than 22 miles the second week, 24 miles the third week, and so on.

- You can proficiently run race pace for a distance equal to three times the length of your average daily run. For example, if you're running 20 miles a week, your daily average is 3 miles, so you can successfully run a race of 9 miles.

- Run three consecutive months of 60 to 70 miles a week to build up a sufficient mileage base to complete a marathon. (This is an axiom to the rule immediately above.)

- Multiply your 10K race time by 4.55 to get your project marathon time (assuming you adhered to the axiom immediately above).

(Another way to predict your marathon time is by using the formula for Yasso 800s, which states your time in minutes and sec-

onds for a workout of 10 times 800 meters—two laps of the track—with equal recovery time being the same as the hours and minutes of your marathon time.)

- Target an even split for both halves of a marathon, but you should realistically expect to run five to seven minutes slower for the second half.

- Expect to lose 1% of your speed every year after you reach 40 years of age.

OK, so far you veterans haven't learned one single thing. Everything you read from this point forward is specifically for you. It's called Ludwig's Third Rule, and it goes something like this:

Once you reach the age of 60, expect all of the numbers you remember from your prime to be adjusted by one-third.

Brace yourself, old-timers, because things are about to get real, if not downright ugly. Here goes:

- If you ran 36-minute 10Ks in your prime, once you become a sexagenarian you'll need to give it everything you've got to run 6.2-miles in 48 minutes, or one-third (12 minutes) slower.

- If you ran three-hour marathons in your prime, you should now expect to run a marathon in four hours, or one-third (one hour) longer.

- If you ran 90-mile weeks in your prime, 60 miles a week (one-third less) will require the same amount of effort once you turn

60. It will also take you the same amount of time it took to run 90 miles in your prime. (See entry immediately below.)

- If you remember what a 7:45-mile training pace in your prime felt like at the time, now a 10:20-mile pace will feel the same.

I told you it was going to be ugly, real ugly.

One last thing: If you're still going (reasonably) strong once you turn 60, you're well on your way to living a long life. In all probability you can expect to live to be well over 80, which if nothing else will prove one thing:

Ludwig's Third Rule might not apply to age.

Let's hope not.

Can I get an Amen?

THE OTHER FOOT

JUNE 2016

"You need to run in these shoes. They're the best!"

"You're crazy if you don't buy a pair of these. Nothing else compares."

"Running shoes will soon be a thing of the past; everyone will be wearing these."

Blah, blah, blah. What works for one person does not always work for another. Remember: It's a little bit different when the shoe is on the other foot.

But since we're on the subject, here's my two cents on the running shoe industry. (Please note: Two cents = the worth of my advice or .015% of what you'll need to buy a new pair of running shoes.) Considering I've worn out well over 100 pairs of running shoes (and counting) in my lifetime, I believe I'm qualified.

- Shoes worthy of your time and money: New Balance, Brooks, Adidas, Saucony, Asics…companies that put the well-being of runners at the forefront.

- Shoes not worthy of your time and money: The company with the "swoosh." Just don't do it; running is now on their back-burner and has been for years. Also anything that resembles what a clown would wear on their feet.

Speaking of things for your feet not worthy of your time and money…

- Many years ago there was an episode of *The Munsters* when Herman, the head of the household (picture a huggable 6'4" Frankenstein's monster) went golfing. When he stepped onto the first putting green, his size-20 boots made 6-foot-deep impressions on the green. Those same size-20 oversized boots with the three-inch heels are now known as Hoka's.

- There is a running shoe that many prominent, world-class runners have had success wearing. I, neither prominent nor world class, can tell you what they did for me: After running in them for a 5-kilometer race both of my shins felt like they had been beaten with a baseball bat. So, you may be asking yourselves, are the shoes any good? Sketchy at best, if you get my drift.

- There are now gloves for your feet. They are to the running industry what eight-track cassette players were to the music industry.

- How about socks with individual compartments for every single one of your toes? They're supposed to reduce the chance of getting blisters on your feet. Since every toe rubs up against a part of the sock, it seems to me they would do just the opposite. I tried putting a pair of them on my feet once. It took me a good seven or eight minutes to put on one sock (each toe has its own slot, and that slot may or may not conform to the size/shape of your toe).

- Trail running shoes. Not that trail running shoes aren't well made and perhaps worthy of their steep price tag; I simply don't believe running and trails are a good fit. I have scars, numbness, and nightmares to support my belief.

- Remember when running barefoot was the thing to do? (Note: It still may very well be in some circles. Don't know; care even less.) Do you remember Zola Budd, the young woman who ran barefoot in the 1984 Summer Olympics? She ran in my running club's Peachtree City 25K several years ago, winning the race and setting a course record in the process. She wore a pair of running shoes.

Finally, one last thing for you to consider:

- Running sandals! I wore them to run all of the downhills at the Badwater Ultramarathon in 2003 to save my toenails from the repeated hammering they would have experienced had I been wearing regular running shoes.* As an added bonus, they're great to wear after any race that beats and badgers your feet beyond recognition.

So, with all of these options and opinions out there, how do you select the right pair of shoes for you?

My advice is to listen.

And I don't mean to listen to the sales staff at your local running shoe store or the person you run with every Saturday morning.

Listen to your feet.

---

* *As for the running shoe I wore at Badwater, I alternated three pairs of New Balance 828s (the best running shoe ever made, in my opinion). I miss them terribly. True story. The end.*

After all (to paraphrase from a slogan used by the "swoosh" company years ago):

Toes know.

I'M NOT SUPERMAN

JULY 2016

I'm writing this for me. I'm sharing it with you because one day—maybe today, maybe 30 years from now—it's worth knowing.

Right now it's important for me, as a long-time runner, to realize I'm not invincible. No one is.

This will serve as my constant reminder.

It's already been 10 days, but it seems like a lifetime ago. Ten days ago something happened to me that having been a runner since the age of 23 I would have never expected.

I had a heart attack.

July 20, 2016. I woke up with a back pain from hell. Somehow, I begged, borrowed, and stole four early morning miles before work. The pain subsided throughout the day until it returned with a vengeance right after lunchtime, only this time the pain was in my chest, and it came back twice as fierce. It wasn't long before I was in a hospital emergency room surrounded by a half-dozen people wearing green coats with stethoscopes around their necks telling me I was having a heart attack.

How could this be? Don't they know I'm a *runner?* I ran my first marathon months after I laced up a pair of running shoes for the first time! My first 50-miler three years after that...my first 100-miler six years after *that!* Perhaps you didn't hear me the first time: I. AM. A. *RUNNER!* You must have me mistaken for someone else. *Runners don't have heart attacks!*

I've run Comrades. I've run JFK. I've run Badwater. I've run Western States. Certainly if I was going to have a heart attack I would have had it by now. These races were in the some of the most demanding conditions imaginable: scorching hot deserts, challenging mountain terrains, and seemingly endless miles. I recovered nicely from all of them, thank you very much. It's what runners do. Now I'm a decade removed from those types of runs; if I were going to have a heart attack certainly I would have had it by now. You must be mistaken. *I don't have heart attacks!*

My resting pulse is 50. I can eat anything I want and not gain a pound. I can survive on five hours sleep a night; I've done it for almost 40 years. My blood pressure is *always* 120/80. When I was 58 a neurologist told me I had the spine of a 30-year-old. *I don't have heart attacks!*

Eight days ago the cardiologist released me from the hospital. He asked me to take it (really, really) easy for six weeks. He imposed a 20-pound lifting restriction on my left arm and a 5-pound restriction on my right arm for five days (he performed a catheterization on that one). I could return to work the following Monday if I worked shorter hours and, as he said before, took it easy.

Monday morning I woke up at my usual time (3 a.m.) and covered four really easy miles. I must have missed the part about staying away from inclines (my wife reminded me of that later) because I was huffing and puffing as I made my way out of my hilly subdivision. When I got home from work I did three more miles on the treadmill. Seven miles and six hours of work on my first day back; why not? After all, *I'm a runner!*

Six days later the five-pound restriction was lifted from my right arm. I figured it was OK to work out with a 40-pound barbell. Why not? Twenty pounds with my left arm plus 20 pounds with my right equals 40 pounds, right? And after all, *I'm a runner!*

Nine days after my heart attack I did five easy miles in the morning, worked six hours, did some shopping on my way home, and then some woodwork for about three hours before calling it a day. Why not, I felt great, and besides, *I'm a runner!*

This morning, 10 days removed from my heart attack, I feel like anything *but* a runner. I woke up feeling like I've been run over by a truck and beyond that have a dull ache in my chest. Thankfully my blood pressure is acceptable or I just might belong in the emergency room again. Apparently being a runner doesn't make me different; it simply makes me human, just like anyone else.

I've got to stop thinking that being a runner gives me superpowers or makes me invincible. Believe me, it doesn't. *Note to self: Please slow down and smell the roses. It would be nice to have you around for another 30 or 35 years.*

Things might be different if I were 31, 41, or, hell, even 51. But I'm not. I'm 61. It's time to grow up.

After all I'm not Superman. Besides, even Superman wasn't invincible; he still had his kryptonite.

As for me, I've got kryptonite of my own: Believing that being a runner makes me invincible.

Take my word for it: It doesn't

FOOL IN THE RAIN

AUGUST 2016

The boys in the lobby of the movie theater looked outside and saw the man in his 20s running in the rain—a rain so cold that it eventually turned into hail. The boys laughed among themselves and reminded one another to slap each other silly if they ever did anything as stupid as wear shorts and run in the cold, cold rain. If the boys had only known the man had just learned he was going to be a father for the first time, they may not have been so judgmental. After all, the young man was a runner, and that's what runners do when they can't find words to express their joy. They run.

The elderly couple sitting on their front porch so they could enjoy the afternoon thunderstorm was caught by surprise when they saw a man in his 30s sprinting past their front yard. They wondered if he was trying to outrun the thunder and lightning and why he didn't have the sense to simply stop and seek shelter. Had they asked, the man would have told them he received a promotion at work earlier in the day, and the run was one of celebration and that he hadn't really noticed he was in the midst of a rain storm. After all, the man was a runner, and that's what runners do when they have something to celebrate. They run.

The kids on the school bus looked outside the window and pressed their faces to the cold glass to see the two men—both in their 40s—running on the side of the road in the middle of a driving snowstorm that was leaving hidden patches of ice in its wake. *Look at the dummies running in the ice and snow!* was a sentiment everyone—including the bus driver—shared as they made fun of the two men. If the occupants of the school bus had only known that one of the runners had cancer, would be gone before the spring thaw, and this was the last time the two of them would run together, they may have felt differently. After all, the men were runners, and that's what runners do when they need to cope. They run.

The newlyweds looked out their front window and saw him. A man—probably in his 50s—running down the street in a torrential downpour. The newlyweds looked at one another, their facial expressions showing they shared the same thought: *Only a fool would be out running on a day like this.* The newlyweds never did take the time to acquaint themselves with the man in his 50s. If they had, they would have learned that he lost his father earlier that day, and the best way of coping with his loss was to go for a run. After all, the man was a runner, and that's what runners do when they need to grieve. They run.

No one saw the man in his 60s as he ran up and down the streets of town at 5 a.m. on a Saturday morning in November in weather that wasn't fit for man or beast. Cold, windy, monsoon-like rain with frequent bursts of thunder and lightning didn't deter the man from his morning run. After all, the man was a runner, and he was simply enjoying something he'd enjoyed doing for almost 40 years. That's what runners do. They run.

It's a shame no one saw the man that morning. For if they had, they would have been able to say they had seen a man who took pride in being known as the fool in the rain.

CLEAN UNDERWEAR

SEPTEMBER 2016

I'm sure I'm not the first child whose mother said to them: *"Always put on clean underwear...just in case you get hit by a bus."* I trust I won't be the last, either. Not to be hit by a bus, but to hear that erstwhile advice.

But the advice hit home recently when I was hit by a bus. Well, I wasn't actually hit by a bus, but I may as well have been because I ended up in the hospital just the same. That sort of thing happens when you have a heart attack, but I'm happy to report that I was in fact wearing a pair of clean underwear at the time. My mom would have been proud; worried out of her mind, of course, but proud.

Today, seven weeks after that eventful day, I'm doing quite well, thank you. Now if I could only get everyone to stop treating me like I'm made of glass, things would be even better.

"You better scale back on your running—have you considered riding a bike?"

"Are you sure eating that rather large bowl of vanilla ice cream is a good idea?"

"You better not try to move that piece of furniture by yourself; here, let me do it for you."

As I said, made of glass.

But when death looks you in the eye and dares you to keep doing the things you've always done—running for hours on end, celebrating Florida Gator touchdowns with a beer, playing with your grandson like there's no tomorrow—it makes you take a step back and give your life choices some serious thought. Thoughts like running 20 miles on Sunday as you've done for the past 20 years might not be such a good idea...or toning down the beer drinking because the Gators are scoring touchdowns like they're going out of style...or taking a step back and letting your grandson expend his energy with his friends rather than you.

After all, I'm getting up in years, and maybe the heart attack was nature's way of telling me to slow down...take it easy...move over to the right side of the road. Besides, slowing down and playing it safe would pretty much assure me of always having on a clean pair of underwear.

But that's the problem. What good is wearing clean underwear if there's no chance of being hit by a bus? I still *want* to run 20-milers. I still *want* to drink beer when the Gators score. I still *want* to play with my grandson. Before long, my legs will tell me 20 miles is out of the question. Before long, my stomach will tell me it's time to stop drinking beer. Before long, my grandson will outgrow rolling around in the back yard with his G-Pa.

Before long, however, isn't now. Right now I want to do the things I've always enjoyed doing. It's what I do, it's what I know, and most of all it's who I am. Sure, the heart attack was a sign that I should do a better job of listening to my body, something I've never been very good at doing. Sure, the heart attack was a sign that I could be making better decisions when it comes to my diet.

Sure, the heart attack was a sign that it's OK to take it easy every now and then.

But the heart attack wasn't a sign to stop doing the things I've always enjoyed doing. Rather, it was a sign that I should be a little more sensible, a little more responsible, and a little more relaxed in the manner I go about things. I'm fine with all of that.

But I'm still alive and kicking and hope to be until the day I die. After all, what's the use of wearing clean underwear if there's virtually no chance of getting hit by a bus?

Besides, if I gave up the things I enjoy, I may as well not wear any underwear at all.

And nobody wants that.

IF I DID RUN

Following the "trial of the century" in which OJ Simpson was found to be not guilty of murdering two people, he wrote a book, If I Did It. It is an alleged fictional account of how he would have committed the murders if he in fact had committed them. While it was promoted as a work of fiction, the general public thought otherwise: It was actually a veiled admission of his guilt; a way to flaunt the fact he had gotten away with the crime of the century.

Inspired by OJ's book, the following is a fictional account of how I've managed to keep my consecutive days of running streak alive since the fall of 1979.

More specifically, since my heart attack in July of 2016.

I knew from the very beginning running would turn into an obsession with me. That's just how I am. If I enjoy something I'll go to great lengths to do it, have it, whatever. Running is something I enjoyed from the very first time I ran three miles in the summer of 1978 in Piedmont Park in the heart of Atlanta. A few months later—on November 30, to be exact—I started something that transformed running into the obsession that it is today. I began running every day. Rain or shine, healthy or not, long or short, early or late…it didn't matter, as long as I got my run in. Every. Single. Day.

It wasn't long before I was running longer and longer distances. Running 15, 20, 25 miles became a compulsion. I wanted to run more miles than anyone I knew. Every. Single. Day. Short runs were for wimps; taking a day off was out of the question.

My lust for mileage got so bad I would fabricate the distances I wrote in my running logs—recording fewer miles than I actually ran, just in case my wife checked behind me to make sure I didn't run more than 10 miles when I had the flu or more than 15 miles the day after I ran a marathon since I had been gone most of the day before and needed to spend time on chores around the house or more than 20 miles on Christmas morning so I could be back home in time for our boys to open their presents. It was bad enough I hosted (and ran) a marathon on three different holidays (New Year's Day, Memorial Day, and Labor Day), and I ran the Atlanta Marathon on Thanksgiving; there was no way she was going to let me spend most of Christmas running with my friends on the one day a year I should devote to my family.

How to run a marathon on Christmas morning

1. Wake up one hour earlier than normal for a 20-mile run. The only one in the house awake will be you.

2. Run 26.2 miles, like you always do on Christmas morning.

3. Return home at the same time you would ordinarily return from a 20-miler, or about the time your wife is waking up and an hour or so before the boys wake up.

I guess I've probably sacrificed four- to five-hundred miles over the past 20 years by "downsizing" the mileage I actually ran. Here are a few examples:

Wife: How far did you run this morning? You said you needed to rest today because you had a long day at work yesterday and would be too tired to help me with the boys' homework tonight.

Me: 7 miles. (Truth: 11 miles.)

Wife: You ran 10 miles this morning. Why did you run again when you got home from work?
Me: I ate a candy bar at work this afternoon and wanted to run it off, so I just did three miles. (Truth: Six miles. And no candy bar.)

Wife: You're sick as a dog and should be going to the doctor. Tell me you didn't run your usual 12 miles this morning.
Me: I didn't. (Truth: 15 miles. And I was actually *sicker* than a dog.)

In all of these cases—and these are just the tips of the iceberg—I recorded in my running logs what I said, not what I actually ran. Believe me: Those four- to five-hundred miles I mentioned earlier is a conservative estimate. The price to keep the peace, I guess.

I've made it clear—on more than one occasion—that the only way I'd end my streak was either through death, being comatose, or because of the loss of a limb (legs only). That being said I knew there would come a time (actually that time has come more than once) when I would be given orders by a doctor to either restrict myself to walking or to not run altogether. As for the former, I've expressed agreement and understanding in the presence of the doctor...and then went home and ran anyway. As for the latter, I simply found myself a new doctor who didn't speak of such nonsense.

Fortunately for me I found a general practitioner who was himself a long-distance cyclist. He understood what running long distances meant to me...what running every day meant to me...what foolishness it was to suggest that I not run. Regardless of what ailment he was treating me for, the last thing he would say to me was to run gently and listen to my body. I always complied, and we got along just fine. I remember having a stress fracture in my left shin and wearing an air cast for about five days. Every afternoon after work I would walk a mile in the air cast, take it off, and head into the woods for an hour or so of running before returning to put the cast back on and walk home.

The United States Running Streak Association has this to say about what constitutes a run:

Run at least one mile (1.61 kilometers) within each calendar day. Running may occur on either the roads, a track, over hill and dale, or on a treadmill.

There was some debate a while back about whether or not walking a mile counted as a run. The arguments went back and forth, and to be honest I wasn't interested enough to stick around to see how things turned out because I was going to run that mile every day, come hell or high water. That way—regardless of the eventual outcome of this great debate—I would be covered. I did tell my friends and family that walking counted toward the continuation of a streak.

I privately called it my insurance policy. But then my GP retired, and as fate would have it that's when I had my heart attack.

During my morning run on July 20, 2016, I was in excruciating pain. Had the pain not been in my back I would have thought— as I mentioned to Cindy before I left the house for my morning run—I was having a heart attack. Somehow, I managed to run four miles—four very, very painful miles—before returning home and getting ready for work. After my shower the pain subsided, and for most of the day I felt OK until mid-afternoon when the pain returned, although this time in my chest. Long story short: I went to the emergency room and was diagnosed as having a heart attack—one I'd been having all day long—and would need a catheterization the following day. As I was rolled into my room in ICU for the night I wondered how I was going to get my run in when I woke up the next morning, confined to a hospital bed, and hooked up to an IV and all sorts of electrical monitors.

Around 5 a.m. I was getting pretty anxious about what the day had in store for me. How long would the catheterization take? Would I get the results and need surgery? Would I still be confined to a hospital bed? WOULD I BE ABLE TO GET MY RUN IN? As I said, I was pretty anxious. In a mild panic, I lifted my legs in the air and started peddling as if I were riding a bicycle. I figured if I did it for 15 minutes I could consider it the equivalent of running a mile "over hill and dale," whatever that means. But after five minutes my stomach was cramping and I was exhausted, thus extending my anxiety over the potential end of my streak.

The catheterization turned out to be a pretty simple procedure; simple for me anyway because I was unconscious the entire time. The results were favorable, as the doctor decided my heart would naturally heal itself and the medications he prescribed would take care of the rest. There was one caveat: No running for six weeks. Later in the day I asked if I could walk the hallways after dinner. He said he didn't see any harm in that. Later that night my friend Valerie came by to see me, and the two of us walked up and down the hallway for 25 minutes—enough time for me to say I covered a full mile. Valerie and Cindy asked me if my streak was still alive, and I told them yes; walking counted. The truth of the matter is I don't know how the debate turned out or if walking did indeed count in the world of running streaks.

But that didn't matter, because earlier that evening I had already run a mile. Let me explain: (1) The nurses told me I couldn't get out of bed to use the restroom. They failed to mention I couldn't get out of bed for any other reason. (2) The doctor already told me I could go for a walk. (3) I ran the day before while I was experiencing a heart attack, so I figured there couldn't be much harm in me running after the heart attack had come and gone. So after dinner and without anyone in the room, I got out of bed, grabbed the rolling cart holding everything I was hooked up to, and ran back in forth in my room for a good 45 minutes. While the pace was anything but fast, I figured I easily covered three miles doing 20-yard fartleks between the door and the window that overlooked the parking lot.

For public consumption I had been seen walking a mile in the halls to keep the streak alive. I couldn't bear for those close to me—family and friends—to think my streak was over or that I would disobey doctor's orders and do anything other than walk. However, behind closed doors I ran three miles to do the same.

One of the benefits of running at oh-dark-thirty every morning is that you do it all alone. I see the occasional car or two, but I seldom see anyone on foot, let alone anyone I know. That is also one of the benefits of walking at that time, so if I were to jog a mile or two when I should be walking no one would know. So every day for those six weeks when I was asked if I ran, I said "certainly not." My thought balloon finished the sentence by adding two more words: "very much." One of the benefits of having the insurance policy I mentioned earlier. The streak lives, and for the time being, so do I.

Postscript: The first day of my official doctor's release to resume running was September 1. On September 5 I ran 15.5 miles (25 kilometers) at my annual Labor Day race. About the time I finished Cindy showed up to walk with her friend Jan. Valerie, whom I ran the 15.5 miles with, told them how far I had run. I've known Cindy since 1973, and I can honestly say I have never seen her that mad. Jan (did I mention she was a nurse?) was right behind her; between the two of them you would have thought I had done something really, really bad.

Like OJ.

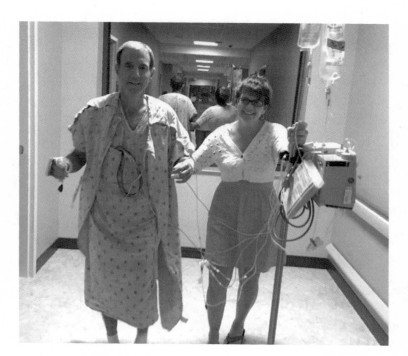

Scott and Valerie, the day after

CREATING A MONSTER

OCTOBER 2016

I've had the opportunity to run with quite a few people in my life, some for too many miles and practically too many years to count. Several have had considerable success, and it always makes me feel good thinking that in some small way I may have played a part in it; I know they have in mine. Don't get me wrong: I am not a coach in any sense of the word. If you ask me about what shoes I wear, how many miles I run, what races I like, or my opinion on all things running, I'll tell you. But one thing I won't do is tell you what *you* should do; that would be your call. Everyone is different: What works for one person may not work for another.

Some of my running companions through the years have gone on to do some rather amazing things:

Kelly Murzynsky, who used to run me into submission on our Sunday morning 20-milers when it was just her and me (and not the rest of the usual suspects) won the first four 50-kilometer ultras she ran.

Valerie Howard, whom I still run with every Saturday and Sunday morning, qualified for the Boston Marathon in 1993 (and would ultimately run 12 of them), competed for the Atlanta Track Club Women's Competitive Team, and served as president of the Atlanta Track Club.

Susan Lance, who won the women's master title at the prestigious Strolling Jim 40-mile run in 2007 and one year later won the overall women's championship. Also in 2008 Susan won a 24-hour treadmill competition by running 108 miles, beating not only the individual entrants, but also the relay teams in the competition; completed the Western States Endurance Run; and won the Lean Horse 100-Mile Run, setting a (then) course record.

Ferit Toska, who was a graduate student at the University of Florida when I met him after speaking at a race expo in Gainesville in 2008, won the Tallahassee Ultra Distance Classic 50-mile run three consecutive years (2013-2015)—quite an accomplishment for someone who was running in soccer shoes the first time I ran with him.

Paula May, who was my crew chief at the Badwater Ultramarathon in 2003 and at one time was one of the fastest grand master's women runners in the southeast while competing for the Atlanta Track Club Women's Competitive Team.

Al Barker, whom I've run more miles with than anyone else, is still enjoying the sport as much as he did when he first started running over four decades ago. I always brag on Al as being the only person I know who has a résumé that includes a sub-five-minute mile, a sub-three-hour marathon, a sub-24-hour 100 miles (at the age of 60, no less), and over 100 marathon finishes. He is also part of two world-record performances—the men's masters 100 x 1-mile relay and the men's grandmasters 100 x 1-mile relay—and was a member of my Badwater crew.

Kelly, Valerie, Susan, Ferit, Paula, Al...they're all amazing athletes who put in a lot of effort and a lot of miles over the years to achieve what they've accomplished. The credit is all theirs, because what drives them comes from within. You've either got it or you don't, and believe me when I tell you this: They are a rare breed, and they have definitely got it. I thought at this point in my life I would never cross paths with another like them.

Then I met Antonio Parks.

Well, I actually met Antonio more than 15 years ago when we worked together for another company. Antonio and I were on the championship mixed volleyball team for a couple of years. He knew I was a runner, but he showed no interest in being one himself.

That all changed a little over six months ago. Having been a volunteer at many of my running club's races over the past several years, Antonio developed an interest in running himself and a little over six months ago asked me for a beginning training plan for runners. I told him what I had done when I started many years ago: Cover two miles a day, running until you had to walk to catch your breath, and then run some more. Just make sure to cover those two miles a day.

In two weeks' time he was up to four miles a day; in four weeks he was up to six. Six weeks into his running career, Antonio ran 26.6 miles at an 8-hour race, his first marathon (and ultra!). His original goal for the event was to run, walk, or crawl 13 miles.

One month later Antonio was joining Valerie and me on Sundays for our long run, usually no less than 14 miles. One month after that he was joining us on Saturdays as well for our other long run of the weekend.

I saw things in Antonio that reminded me of me almost 40 years ago. A fascination with the many different models of running shoes (although to be fair, Antonio has a larger variety to obsess over than I did), a keen interest in learning about what he should and shouldn't be doing in his training, and a zealousness to get out and run usually seen in someone 20 (if not 30) years his junior.

As he did at last year's Senoia 60—a two-and-a-half-day event in which participants complete as many miles as they can—Antonio and his friend Ken Menefield volunteered to staff the aid station, counting laps, refilling water coolers, keeping the restrooms clean, for the duration of the event. At this year's Senoia 60 he not only volunteered to count everyone's miles, but he also racked up 109 of his own.

Leading up to the event he was just hoping to get in a run on all three days (Friday, Saturday, and Sunday). Before long he was feeling confident he was capable of running as much as 50 miles. Later he upped the ante to a marathon a day. So when Antonio and I were running one of the 6.5-mile loops on Saturday and I told him he was already at 50 miles and there were still 30 hours left, I could tell by the look on his face that he had a new goal in mind: 100 miles. Remember, this is a man who had only been running a little more than six months.

As he was approaching 100 miles Antonio told me if he got there he would definitely stop running. I knew better. In fact I told him so: *"No you won't."* You know the rest.

I've had the good fortune of having many Antonio's in my life. It keeps me going, and to be quite honest Antonio couldn't have come along at a better time. I'm slowing down and certainly not getting any younger, and yes, there are even days when running is more pain than pleasure, but Antonio—and many others before him—always seem to come into my life at just the right time to keep the fire burning.

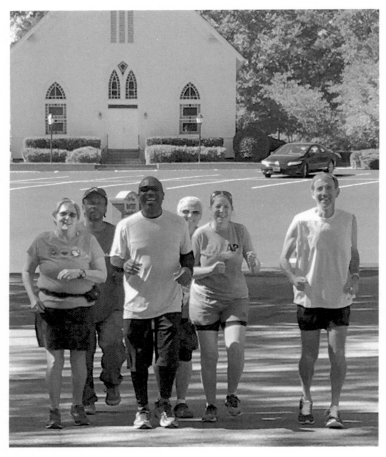

Antonio (front and center) completing his first 100-miler in Senoia, Georgia

STRESS TEST

OCTOBER 2016

The heart attack had been over three months ago. My follow-up appointment with the cardiologist was still two weeks away. I wanted to see for myself how I was doing.

That's my story, and I'm sticking to it.

I decided to compete in the Senoia 60, an event designed for runners to compile as many miles as they can in a 60-hour window that starts Friday morning and ends Sunday night. Being the race director of the event I was going to be there anyway, so why not put in a few miles while I was there?

My wife Cindy asked me not to overdo it. I promised I wouldn't and that I'd take it easy, very easy. I stayed true to my words except those two times when I was running alone and I heard someone coming up beside me and that old instinct to *not let anyone pass me under any circumstance* kicked in (they didn't, by the way).

In all honesty, the hard part of the weekend was getting everything set up for the event (marking the course, setting up the aid station, putting out signage) and then of course cleaning everything up. The running was the easy part.

By 10 p.m. on the first day I had completed 50 miles. In my mind I started the event thinking I had plenty of time over the course of the weekend to reach 100 miles. I decided to wait until after a few hours of sleep to see how I felt.

My goal for the second day was not to do anything that would make me want to exceed what I ran last year (152 miles). I took it easy through lunchtime, left in the afternoon to attend a neighborhood block party (Note: I had a great reason for leaving the party before it was over: I was in the middle of a race.), played host to "Senoia Rick," a lookalike for Rick Grimes, the main character in the popular television series *The Walking Dead,* ran a couple of miles with my grandson (he said he loved running in the dark for the first time, although I think it was because he had a blast shining my flashlight in everyone's face), before calling it a day (literally and figuratively) at midnight. By then I had another 43.5 miles under my belt.

I went home and slept for about four hours and woke up the third day a bit sore; the kind of sore that works its way out of your body after running for 45 minutes. Up until this point the only thing Cindy asked me the three or four times she saw me was *"you're not overdoing it, are you?"* Each time I asked her to look at me and decide if I looked like I was. I passed the test each time. Fortunately she never asked about my mileage, not once. My guess is it was intentional because she didn't really want to know.

That is, until she came by Sunday night as the race was drawing to a close. She picked up the clipboard and saw "82.0" at the bottom of the page with my name on it. Sarcastically and a bit condescendingly, she said, *"82 miles...REALLY?"*

---

*   *Many of the scenes from the show were filmed in the area we were running. Senoia Rick works on weekends, giving Walking Dead tours. He is a dead ringer for Rick Grimes, and the runners familiar with the show enjoyed his visit.*

In the most innocent voice I could muster I said, *"I don't know—I wasn't keeping up with it."* At the same time I was praying she wouldn't look over at the second column and see the final number recorded on my page: 119.0. (She never did.)

It seems that everything is working, and I'm well on the road to recovery. In a couple of weeks I'll go see the cardiologist, so he can tell me what I already know.

I have no intention of telling him about those 119 miles. He just wouldn't understand.

I will tell him there's no need for me to take a stress test, though. That ship has sailed.

TURKEY DAY

NOVEMBER 2016

It was just after 8 a.m. the Saturday before Thanksgiving. Valerie and I were 10 miles into our run when we noticed several wild turkeys mixing it up with some chickens in the yard of a house on one of the country roads in Senoia. We stopped to catch a glimpse of the action when suddenly the turkeys started running along the 100-yard asphalt driveway toward the road we were standing on. Jokingly I mentioned to Valerie that the turkeys were coming after us. Thirty seconds later I discovered the joke was on me.

Because 30 seconds is how long it took for five of the largest and loudest turkeys I've ever run across to take their position between Valerie and me, frozen in our tracks as we both wondered what was about to happen. Valerie spoke up first: *"They're going to dance for us."* (She explained later she used to have a turkey— Tom Turkey—who would dance in circles whenever she was around.) We waited a few seconds; dancing was the last thing on their minds. I looked up and down the street, hoping for someone to open their front door and reassure us they were neighborhood turkeys who wouldn't do us any harm, throw some bird food from their front porch to distract them, or at least tell us they had called 911. None of that happened.

Valerie and I watched the turkeys intently while they watched intently back. The tallest one—whose head came up to my chest and probably weighed at least five pounds of feathers more than me— was the loudest…and meanest looking of the lot. Don't get me wrong: Any one of the others would be enough to cause concern if you met up with them in a dark alley. After five or six minutes of gobbling, flapping their wings, ruffling their tail feathers, circling and intermittently creeping toward Valerie (and her two dogs who had been running with us) and me, the turkeys maintained their proximity to us. I looked at Valerie and said "checkmate" because I felt like we were in the middle of a Mexican standoff, except with wild turkeys and no guns. (My best guess is that during this time the turkeys were wondering whether or not we were carnivores. Truth be told I was wondering the exact same thing about *them.*)

As both my eyes were focused on the turkeys and what they might do next, I failed to notice that Valerie and her dogs were slowly distancing themselves from me and our feathered friends. I looked up and saw Valerie and her dogs were almost 40 yards away while the turkeys were still hovering in front of me, never more than a couple of feet apart and always forming a perfect circle. All I could think of was this:

I have to make a run for it.

So I did. I ran toward Valerie, slowly at first just to see what the turkeys would do. They ran after me, keeping their distance at a couple of yards. I wasn't sure if they were enjoying the run or were trying to catch me and peck me to the ground. I ran faster; they did the same. I ran even faster, so did they. Finally I broke out in a full sprint and gave it everything I had. I looked back and saw I had finally managed to open up a little distance between the turkeys and me, and I started to breathe easier when I saw them stop dead in their tracks in the middle of the road. *(A quick calculation: Turkeys max out at about seven minutes per mile, based solely on when this particular gang decided to call it quits.*

Interesting fact: A group of wild turkeys is called a flock, whereas a group of domesticated turkeys is known as a gang. Backwards, I know. During my research I also discovered turkeys can run 25 miles per hour. I'm glad I did this research after my escape from danger; otherwise I just might have wet my shorts.)

I regret Valerie didn't have a cell phone with her so she could take a photograph; I can only imagine what I looked like running as fast as I could with five rather large wild turkeys in close pursuit. I have no idea what the expression on my face was because it was a blend of deathly fear, reaching my anaerobic threshold, disbelief, and the slightest hint of a smile, because I knew that in a million years nothing like this would never happen again.

I was also proud of myself for proving an old adage to be entirely false, because regardless of what anyone says you *can* fly like an eagle when you're surrounded by turkeys.

GROSS

DECEMBER 2016

I recently ran my 144,000th lifetime mile. If mileage was packaged into 12,000-mile bundles, I'd have a gross* of them.

That's quite a bit when I think about it. It's almost six laps around the earth, it's over halfway to the moon, and it would take light almost a full second to travel that far. Not bad for a 62-year-old pair of legs that hasn't seen a day of rest since 1978.

Gee, you must be tired. No and yes. No, because every morning I still have whatever energy is needed to put in 60 to 65 miles a week out on the roads. Yes, because every night I have no problem falling asleep in my lounge chair before the sun goes down (even in the winter when it's dark by 5:30!). If you listen to my wife, if I didn't wake up every morning at 3 a.m. to run I would have more energy at night and wouldn't need to be in bed early enough to get in my requisite 5.5 hours of sleep. But when you have a full-time job and enough part-time hobbies to account for every waking moment (not to mention a grandson I'll drop whatever I'm doing to spend time with), getting enough sleep is not really an option.

Besides, running has given me a lot of joy through the years and seems to have been doing a pretty good job of keeping those extra holiday pounds at bay. So every year I convince myself to make a change the following year that allows me more time to sleep, and every year I get the same result. Nothing changes.

---

*   *Gross (noun) – an amount equal to twelve dozen*

To be totally honest it's hard to change things up when you have a gross of miles in your back pocket. Running that far and for that long (38 years and counting) has a way of defining a person. It's difficult to change who you are and what makes you happy.

Of course I could try focusing on those moments when running caused me a lot of pain, discomfort, and misery. For example:

- After running 159 miles in three days in my initial attempt (a failure, as I was 121 miles shy of my goal) at running across the state of Georgia in 1982, I was forced to run in an air cast for a week while my stress fracture in my left shin healed.

- At the 2000 Shamrock Marathon (mile 20, I remember it oh so well) I turned a corner and felt something snap in my right thigh. The numbness I felt that day still remains, 16-plus years later.

- At the 2004 Western States Endurance Run I injured my back running up and down mountains for 62 miles. I had never run mountains like that before and had no idea what I was getting myself into. I have back issues to this day.

- At the 2006 Western States I literally shred the bottoms of my feet after running in soaking wet shoes for the better part of 100 miles. I hobble-ran for several weeks after that as my feet mended ever so slowly.

There were a lot more, of course, but these are the first four that came to mind. And you get the idea.

Then again, I could have simply included a photograph of the bottoms of my feet after Western States.

But I decided against it. That would just be gross.*

---

*   *Gross (adjective) – disgusting, offensive, vulgar*

62*

JANUARY 2017

I can see by the look on your face you're confused by the title of this story. Baseball aficionados may be thinking it's a reference to me hitting 62 home runs in a 154-game season of major league baseball; you know, similar to how Roger Maris' homerun total in 1961 is frequently notated (61*). If that's the case you would be sadly mistaken. Following is a summary of my entire baseball career. See for yourself:

I played organized baseball for one season. It was the summer of 1966, the longest summer of my life. I was 11 years old and played right field for the Douglasville (Rhode Island) Wolves. Each game consisted of me standing in right field for four or five minutes, then sitting on the bench for four or five minutes for seven innings, and two or three times a game grabbing a bat and standing at home plate trying not to get hit by a 55-mile-per-hour pitch thrown by another 11-year-old with absolutely no business whatsoever throwing a baseball in my general vicinity.

As you might infer, I never hit 62 home runs in a season.

But I have run 62 miles. Many times, actually. And not once did I have to dodge a baseball coming at me at 55 miles per hour. A beer bottle thrown at my head by a driver obviously under the influence maybe, but never have I had to dodge a fastball while out for a run.

Enough about my baseball career; let me get back to the title and explain what it means.

For all 38 calendar years (1979-2016) I have completed during my consecutive-days running streak, I have averaged at least as many miles per week as the age I reached during that year.

But that streak will end in 2017. I'm certain of it.

2016 was difficult, to say the least. A heart attack on July 20 put a serious dent in my mileage. Somehow, I managed to put in enough time on the asphalt the last four months of the year to finish with an average of 62 miles a week for 2016. I turned 62 on December 10. By December 31 I was so tired that I didn't do what I normally do on the first day of a new year: run lots of miles. (I stopped at 8.)

So to suggest that I can average 63 miles a week—9 miles a day— in 2017 seems a bit far-fetched.

I verified my running logs to double-check my statement of having averaged at least as many miles per week as my age in any given calendar year. I even asked Ernst and Young to count behind me (they refused; they didn't actually refuse, but rather quoted a price to do it that was way out of my ballpark).

But after double-checking here's a few interesting things I ran across:

1980. My lowest weekly mileage ever (34), the result of a knee injury that was so painful I submitted to an injection of cortisone that was even more painful than the knee injury itself. I ran one hour after the injection after the doctor instructed me not to run for a couple of days. It was one of the worst decisions of my running career (getting the injection, not running after I was told not to).

1985. The only other time I averaged 63 miles a week in a year. I turned 31 that year. To put that into perspective, that was over 50% of my life ago.

1986. I averaged 73 miles a week for the year. I ran my marathon PR in January of 1987. When I'm asked how many miles per week someone needs to prepare for a marathon, I always tell them 73. Now you know why. (Note: I was 32 years old when I ran my marathon PR, which according to legend, is the prime age of a marathoner. Maybe legend has it right.)

1994. I averaged 89 miles a week for the year. It was the year I started running with Valerie Howard and Al Barker. This kind of mileage would continue for almost two decades. They are both to blame (don't let them tell you anything different).

1998. I averaged 104 miles a week for the year, my most ever. I ended the year with a win at the Tallahassee Ultra Distance Classic 50K in one of the best races I've ever run. I'm convinced even now I could have continued the pace I ran that day (7:14 per mile) for another 19 miles and won the 50-mile version of the race that day. I turned 44 that year so my weekly mileage exceeded my age by 60, my all-time high.

2006. I averaged 92 miles a week for the year. I mention it because for the last 13 years (1994 through 2006), I averaged 91 miles a week—or 13 miles (a half marathon) per day.

2015. I turned 61 that year. It will turn out to be the last year I averaged 70 miles a week, or 10 miles a day.

Interestingly enough, I calculated my daily average for the duration of my running career and translated it into a weekly average: 73.

However, I doubt my marathon PR is in any sort of jeopardy.

2017

WELL PAST THE FINISH LINE

A SHOULDER TO CRY ON

JANUARY 2017

Ask any long-term runner and they'll all tell you the same thing: Over time a runner will discover two or three fellow runners they can truly count on; someone who will always be there when it's time to go for a run. No matter what, when or where, (and occasionally why), they will always be there for you.

As I've said before, runners are the finest people I've ever met. I've been fortunate to share the roads with quite a few of them over the year. Some have moved away, some are no longer physically able to run, and sadly, some are simply no longer with us.

I still run regularly with a couple of people whom I've run with for many, many years. We've shared many a mile running along too many roads to count in too many places to possibly remember. We've pushed ourselves physically, endured the worst weather imaginable, and experienced virtually every injury under the sun. During all of it, we've no doubt shared every last detail of our lives with each other.

Most of all we've always been there for each other. I'd go as far as saying we confide things to one another that we've never shared with anyone else. Because that's what runners do; they share a special connection that is impossible to explain but universally understood by runners everywhere.

My closest running friends probably know me better than I know myself. That's what happens when you share all of your hopes, dreams, highs, lows, good times, and bad over endless miles and countless hours. I referred to this once as "asphalt therapy," but it's so much more than that.

There will always be times when things aren't going your way or how you would like them to be going. Your partners will be there to listen, offer advice, and provide encouragement. And if necessary they'll lend you a shoulder to cry on.

There may be times, of course, when you'll have to (or may simply want to) run alone, and there won't be anyone there for you to pour your heart out to.

Just remember, the road always has a shoulder for you to cry on.

LOWERING THE BAR

MARCH 2017

I've been running marathons since 1979. In every last one of them I've always had a goal; one that continued to raise the bar higher and higher. Finish. Break three-and-a-half hours. Run through the wall. Break three hours. Qualify for Boston. Set a personal best. Set another personal best…and another.

Later, as age caught up with me and took its toll on my endurance and to an even greater degree my speed, the focus was no longer on raising the bar but rather on making each marathon a memorable one. I'm happy to say that I was never disappointed. It may have been because I was able to run in a new and exciting locale, help another runner achieve a personal goal, or simply meet new people along the way who would ultimately become friends for life.

The past few years the goal has simply been to turn each marathon into an adventure. It's not that any of my marathons haven't been, but rather to say that if that adventure no longer existed the thrill of running a marathon would be lost.

This morning, as I lace up my shoes for a marathon, my goal is simply this: Don't die. After suffering a heart attack a little over seven months ago, I think the goal is realistic. My heart doctor—who has given me a green light to continue running with one caveat, *don't push it*—is in my corner. My friends who I'll be running with today are both in my corner: Val, who I've run marathons with for the past two dozen years, and Antonio, who is

313

running his very first marathon and in all probability will be the last person I'll ever personally have any influence on in becoming a long-distance runner. They as well as I know there is a very real possibility that the thrill of pounding the pavement for most of the morning is also an open invitation for the Grim Reaper to rain at any time on my 26.2-mile parade.

However, at 7 a.m. the three of us stand shoulder to shoulder with 1,000-plus like-minded souls who understand that a healthy life-style is the best method of keeping death at arm's length. Val, Antonio, and I enjoyed the cool, crisp morning running along the streets of Albany, Georgia, to the constant cheers from the local citizens who more than once thanked us for coming to their fair city to run. No, Albany; thank you for having us. By noon Val completed another marathon, bringing her lifetime total to some-where near 100. Antonio successfully finished his first, and by all indications there will be many more to come. As for me, I'm just happy to report I followed my doctor's orders, and it worked: I crossed the finish line, and I didn't die.

I spent a cool, crisp morning running for a very long time with two of my closest running companions in one of the most runner-friendly cities I know. We all finished, and we got together after-ward to celebrate.

I would never have guessed that by setting the bar so low I was actually raising it higher than it's ever been.

Epilogue: It was 38 years ago this month that I ran my very first marathon in Gainesville, Florida. Moments before the start I asked (then) University of Florida running coach Roy Benson for any advice he could offer. His response—I can still hear it to this day—was terse and to the point: *Don't run marathons.* He was being dead serious.

Well Coach, after 200-plus marathons I've decided to take your advice. I can walk away with the knowledge that the bar is resting comfortably on the top rungs.

PODCAST FODDER

MARCH 2017

The other day I was asked to appear on the East Coast Trail and Ultra Podcast by one of the hosts, Ryan Ploeckelman. I asked what we would be talking about. *"Running and sh*t."* I told Ryan he was in luck because I just so happen to do both: One I do every day, and the other I'm lucky if I do every *other* day. Regardless of their respective frequencies, however, I consider myself as an expert on both.

Ryan told me Sean Blanton was the other host of the show. I first met Sean several years ago when he won one of our Darkside holiday marathons in Peachtree City. Sean, or "Run Bum" as he is known in running circles, could be the poster boy for the phrase "free spirit." I have a special respect for Sean because he's done a few runs that remind me of some of the crazy things that I did when I was closer to his age. (Confession time: *I still do them, just not as fast as I used to.*)

As for Ryan, he's got that distinctive disk jockey voice that catches your attention and won't let go. Ryan and Sean complement one another perfectly, and it was evident they had done their homework prior to my interview. Well, *most* of it anyway.

They started the podcast by asking me about my 38-plus years of running every day and that my streak was old enough to legally drink a beer. *Do you remember the last day you didn't run? What made you start your streak? Do you know I wasn't born when you started your streak? Have you ever been injured?* The only question they didn't ask—and I hear it from people all the time—is this: *Don't you feel better after you take a day off?* (Answer: I wouldn't know.) I know they were doing their best asking those questions, but I also know this: I don't enjoy being asked about my streak. That's the homework they failed to do. If you have to ask me about my streak you wouldn't understand, and there's no way in the world I can explain it in such a way that it makes any sense. So if you were planning on asking me about it, there's really no need.

They asked about some of my favorite races, how the Darkside Running Club came to be, and how ultras have changed since the first one I ran in 1995. I corrected them and said my first ultra was in the 80s. They said Ultra Signup (where they found out about my racing history) only dated back to 1995, thus putting an exclamation point on their previous comment about not being born when my streak began. As for how I answered those three questions: (1) I was very fond of the former Vulcan Marathon in Birmingham, particularly the Twinkies and champagne at the 10-mile aid station; (2) Al Barker, four others, and I formed the club officially in 2002, and the membership has grown from an original six members to now over 500 members; and (3) there are so many more 24-hour events now than there were when I was in my prime as well as a lot more interest in trail (as opposed to road) ultras. As for that last answer, there's one other bit of homework Ryan and Sean failed to do. Otherwise they would have known how much I hate trail running and wouldn't have taken the time during my interview to talk about how much *they* enjoyed it. (Note: Don't get me wrong; I respect trail running. I just don't consider it to be true "running." Plus I suck at it. And I fall down. A lot.)

Then again, they may have been baiting me, although I seriously doubt it. They both seem to be really nice guys doing their absolute best to produce a quality product for runners to enjoy.

Better yet, the podcast appears to be a labor of love for them both. I'm guessing when they did their homework, they found out how much things of that nature mean to me.

Which explains why it was a pleasure being on their show.

If you want to hear the podcast in its entirety: East Coast Trail & Ultra, March 16, 2017,

Episode 25: All is Fair on the Trail, Even Cursing a Pastor.

LET IT GO

APRIL 2017

It started out almost as a joke. "The Darkside" as we called ourselves in the mid-1990s when Al Barker, Valerie Howard, and I started running weekly 20-milers so we would be marathon ready year-round. While all the other runners in town were eating pancakes or getting ready for church after their six- or eight-mile Sunday morning runs, the three of us were still on the trails doing what we liked to do best.

In 2002 the three of us, along with Kelly Murzynsky, Paula May, and Sue Bozgoz, decided to form the Darkside Running Club. I was selected (not elected, but selected) to be president. Little did I know at the time the title of president also bestowed upon me the duties of the vice president, secretary, treasurer, newsletter editor, race director, volunteer coordinator, and essentially any other job that needed to be done at any given time.

Over time the club—primarily via word of mouth—took on additional members, and during the winter of 2017 we welcomed our 500th member—or Darksider as we prefer to be called. I always said that when our club membership reached 500 it would be time for a new president, although truth be known I've been searching for a new president for the past two years. Coincidentally, one of our members stepped forward to take over as president at just about the same time we welcomed our 500th Darksider. I'm guessing karma had a little something to do with it.

As of July 1, 2017, Joye McElroy will assume the presidency of the Darkside Running Club. Joye has asked me to stay close in an unofficial capacity to which I agreed…as long as I'm referred to as president emeritus. (Note: I was half kidding when I mentioned it, but when she agreed I thought it sounded sort of cool. So I'm using it. Try and stop me.) Whatever the case, after more than 15 years directing the club I was part of putting together it's going to be a little hard for me to let go. I know what you're thinking: baby steps. That's probably how it will be, and I'm good with that. But it won't be the same.

After directing well over 100 Darkside events, publishing 63 issues (totaling more than 4,000 pages) of absolutely true *Takes from the* DARKSIDE (our quarterly newsletter), and doing everything in my power to promote our running club to the rest of the world, it's going to be quite a change for me to step aside.

I've enjoyed being in the driver's seat all of these years. Welcoming new members into the club, seeing so many runners doing things they never dreamed possible, introducing so many people to the sport of running, and best of all promoting their accomplishments are the things that made being president of the Darkside Running Club so darn rewarding.

I'm proud of what the Darkside Running Club represents: setting your goals high, encouraging and supporting your fellow runners, never giving up or backing down from a challenge, and doing things you always dreamed of doing but never thought possible. Best of all, it's the only running club I know of that essentially pays *you* to be a member. Allow me to explain:

Lifetime dues are $35 per family. There is nothing else to pay to be a member...ever. Any profits the club incurs (primarily through entry fees) are given back to the members through reduced entry fees to Darkside events, occasional stipends for sponsored races, and various other fringe benefits that you'd have to be a member to know about.

I doubt you'll find another running club anything like it. If you do, chances are they borrowed their formula from us.

Here's to many more years of pushing the limits of human endurance and making the impossible possible.

Here's to many more years of the Darkside Running Club.

We're in it for the long run.

WHEN I'M 64

APRIL 2017

Will you still need me, will you still feed me, when I'm sixty-four?
–Paul McCartney and John Lennon

I will celebrate my 64th birthday on December 10, 2018. Originally, I intended for this book to be published on that date, but then decided against it. Here's why:

I'm what you might call a "numbers guy." If I get a number in my head it's easy for me to fixate on that number until it's realized. Once I realized many years ago that running was going to be a lifetime commitment I set three goals for myself: 100,000 miles, 1,000 races, and 100 marathons. While the 1,000 races continue to be a work in progress, the other two goals were accomplished years ago.

So I raised the bar to 150,000 miles and 200 marathons. The 2012 Honolulu Marathon was my 200th and doubled as a 35-year wedding anniversary trip to Oahu for Cindy and me. As for those 150,000 miles...

Remember when I said once I get a number in my head it's easy for me to fixate on that number until it's realized? Remember when I said I originally intended for this book to be published when I turn 64?

2018 could be a big year for me, big in the sense that several of the numbers in my head could very possibly be realized before the year is over. If all goes as planned, I will run my 40th consecutive Peachtree Road Race on July 4, 2018. If all goes as planned, I hope to complete my 40th consecutive year of running every day on November 29, 2018. If all goes as planned, I hope to run my 150,000th lifetime mile on December 10, 2018, my 64th birthday.

As for my original thought to publish this book when I turn 64, that's where I had to draw the line. I didn't want to delay the book simply to coincide with the numbers I had in my head. Let's just say that publishing the book at this time is an honest effort on my part to stop letting numbers play such a large role in my life.

As you can imagine, there's more to my fascination with numbers outside of running. If you asked me to, I could give you enough examples to fill another book, but you'll just have to take my word for it because trust me, you really don't want to know. Or you could just take the 77,642 words in this book for it. *(See how it works?)*

I hope you enjoyed this book. I hope it helps your running. I hope you were able to discern between the things you should be doing and more importantly the things you *shouldn't* be doing.

Most of all, I hope you learned there are more important things in life than the number of marathons and miles you run or how many days, months, or years you run consecutively. For the most part, I learned the hard way.

What's important is that you are a runner and as you know from reading this book:

Runners are some of the finest people I know.

EPILOGUE

READING BETWEEN THE LINES

Following is a condensed summary of what was presented in this book thus far.

Aspiring runners will want to pay close attention.

Grizzled veterans will merely sigh and remember when "those were the days."

Find a reliable partner (or two) to make those long weekend runs more enjoyable.

Don't become obsessed with how many, how long, how far, how fast, etc. I'm here to tell you: Numbers can often be the devil.

Support local running events supporting a worthy cause; ones that offer an affordable entry fee, a safe and well-marked course, supportive volunteers and an appreciative race director.

Don't stress over things outside of your control; bad weather, for example. There's a silver lining in every cloud; look hard enough and you'll find it.

Stay positive and focused. The only thing standing in the way of reaching your goals is you.

If you qualify for the Boston Marathon, by all means: Do everything in your power to be in Hopkinton on Patriot's Day!

Have the good sense to realize when enough is enough.

Streak running is not nearly as glamorous as it sounds. Whatever you do, take a rest day every now and then.

Never start anything you're not prepared to finish.

Finish what you started. If not this time, next time.

Run the Peachtree Road Race at least once in your life. There's nothing like it.

By all means run in the rain. It's exhilarating.

Protect your body from the elements (sun, rain, cold, etc.). It's the only body you have so take good care of it.

Listen to your body. Don't run if you're sick, injured or in dire need of rest.

Stretching is never a bad thing. Neither is lifting weights every now and then.

Don't be intimated by the accomplishments of other runners; rather, be inspired.

Relish the satisfaction of finishing each and every run. Recognize each run as an accomplishment.

Encourage others to be the best runner they can possibly be.

When it's your turn—and you will now when it is—give back to the sport of running.

Don't run your first trail race if the distance is further than 10 kilometers. By no means should your first trail race be 100 miles; the Western States Endurance Run, for example.

Dream big, but don't bite off more than you can chew. Easier said than done.

LISTEN to the veteran runners; they know what they're talking about.

Test drive running shoes before you pay good money for them.

If you run in the dark, wear something that makes you visible to others.

If you decide to participate in a 'big ticket' race, do it for the right reasons. 'Because all the cool kids are doing it' is not one of them.

Running is a sport made for optimists. Pessimists need not apply.

If your running has the support of your family, know that you are blessed. Be grateful.

Recognize when it's time to let go, but know the difference between letting go and giving up.

If people want to know 'all about your running' they will ask. Refrain from telling them about it unless they do.

If you have the chance, pass along the gift of running.

(As much as I hate to admit it) Running is not a clothing-optional sport.

Respect your elders in running; respect your elders in life.

When it comes to running, spend your money wisely. Sadly there are people who are only in the sport to make a buck.

Every marathon should be an adventure. When they cease to be, it's probably time to call it quits.

Accept the fact that some runners just don't have any business running trails. Be aware you may be one of them.

Be sure to read books about running written by Scott Ludwig. You have eight to choose from.

Have the good sense to know when to quit, when to say no and when to say enough is enough.

Contrary to popular belief: You *can* run too much.

Running offers a time to think, a time to plan and a time to relax. Not only that, it's a natural stress reliever and if you haven't heard already, it's pretty good exercise!

Keep your personal accomplishments in perspective. What impresses you may not impress others. The only person you need to impress is you.

Remember what got you this far.

If your spouse or mate supports your running, consider yourself fortunate. If your spouse or mate is a runner, consider yourself one lucky son-of-a-b*tch.

Respect the accomplishments and personal triumphs of other runners.

Remember running does not make you invulnerable. Of all people, I should know.

There is no need to rush back from an injury or an illness. The roads will patiently await your return.

Age gracefully and be content to rest on your laurels when your time comes.

Live every day as if it could be your last. You owe it to your family, your friends, your loved ones and most of all yourself.

The road always has a shoulder for you to cry on.

IN CLOSING

This morning as I was finishing up my run I noticed an armadillo bouncing off the curb every 15 feet or so as it was trying to jump on a yard but couldn't jump high enough to clear the cement.

I was thinking how armadillos must be the dumbest creatures in the world, so out of sympathy I shined my flashlight on a driveway so the armadillo could see the driveway and gain access to a neighbor's yard.

It was at that moment I ran into a garbage can I didn't see because I was using my flashlight to help the armadillo.

Stupid armadillo!

Scott Ludwig
April 20, 2017
Senoia, Georgia

ACKNOWLEDGMENTS

As I read over the manuscript one last time before the book went to print I couldn't help but think how many people through the years have had an impact on what went into these pages. There is no way I could possibly name all of them, but I'm going to try:

If you ever directed or volunteered in a race I've competed in, took the time to read something I've written, joined the Darkside Running Club, supported me in one of my adventures, had the opportunity to listen to me speak, or simply ran a mile or two with me: THANK YOU!

As she has so many times before, Susanne Thurman has provided invaluable assistance in formatting this book and assisting with the photographs. Words couldn't possibly thank her enough for her help (but as I've come to find out, chocolate can).

While all the photographs are from my personal collection, my thanks to those who were on the other side of the camera when they were taken. As for the photos of Krischan after his first race and my bloody body parts after my last trail run (ever), those were taken by yours truly.

The author image on the back cover is a pencil drawing by the very talented JaRodney Anderson and is a recreation of a photo taken of me during the 2006 Shamrock Marathon in Virginia Beach, Virginia. The race holds special meaning to me because it always gave me the opportunity to spend time with my parents when they were still alive and living in nearby Chesapeake. Not a day or a run goes by that I don't think about them.

Finally, the biggest thank you of all goes out to the original Running Widow, my wife Cindy. As I've stated before, she's been with me every step of the way. I just hope there are many more to come.

I may be running on fumes at this point, but I'm still running.

CREDITS

Design and Layout

Cover and Interior Design: Annika Naas
Layout: ZeroSoft

Editing

Managing Editor: Elizabeth Evans

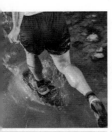

MORE GREAT RUNNING TITLES

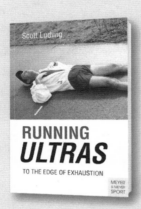

ISBN 9781782550464
352 p., b/w, 23 photos
paperback, 5.5" x 8.25"
$14.95 US

Scott Ludwig

RUNNING ULTRAS

TO THE EDGE OF EXHAUSTION

Running Ultras chronicles the author's journey (the training, the races, and the people he met along the way) to complete his personal quest of running four major ultramarathons: the JFK 50-Mile Run, Badwater Ultramarathon, Western States Endurance Run, and the Comrades Marathon.

FROM MEYER & MEYER SPORT

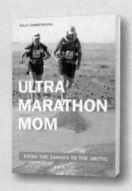

Holly Zimmermann

ULTRAMARATHON MOM

FROM THE SAHARA TO THE ARCTIC

Ultramarathon Mom is the unique story of a mother who ran some of the world's most difficult and dangerous foot races. Forrest-Gump-like happenstances paired with practical tips make this book a must-read for ultrarunners.

ISBN 9781782551393
200 p., b/w, 20 photos
paperback, 5.5" x 8.5"
$14.95 US

MEYER & MEYER Sport
Von-Coels-Str. 390
52080 Aachen
Germany

Phone   +49 02 41 - 9 58 10 - 13
Fax   +49 02 41 - 9 58 10 - 10
E-Mail   sales@m-m-sports.com
Website www.m-m-sports.com

All books available as E-books.

MEYER
& MEYER
SPORT